LEADING
A BALINT GROUP

a Guide

Heide Otten

Psyllabus publishing house
Moscow 2018

*Psyllabus publishing house holds the exclusive
publishing rights for the book by*

Heide Otten
"Leading a Balint group. a Guide"

Translated from English by Anna Tishkova

This book will be interesting and useful for various specialists involved in the practice of Balint group work and willing to obtain a Balint group leader certificate. In a very comprehensible form, it gives an account of the manifold aspects of Balint group leaders' training and work, the types of Balint groups and their main features, as well as what a Balint group is not by definition. The author thoroughly considers the following issues: the leader's position in a Balint group, the co-leader's job, the parallel process, specificity of leaders' training: requirements, stages and criteria. The book tells about styles of leading different groups, eg. homogeneous and heterogeneous groups, groups with physicians, psychologists and psychiatrists as well as with members of other helping professions. The aspects of supervision for Balint group leaders and the key leader's tasks in a classical and sculpture group are also covered. A special Appendix features the main guidelines of the International Balint Federation for accreditation of Balint group leaders and criteria for their accreditation in Germany.

This book is a mutual project of Dr. Heide Otten and Psyllabus publishing house.

© Psyllabus publishing house, 2017
© Heide Otten, 2017
© Anna Tishkova, translation into Russian, 2017
© Sergey Sholkov, illustrations, 2017

ISBN 978-5-6040138-0-9

www.psyllabus.biz

About the author

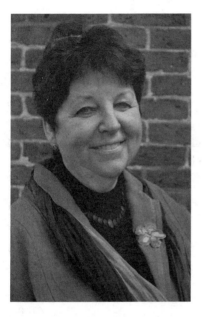

Dr. Heide Otten was born on September 18th, 1944 in Germany. From 1964-1970 she attended medical school in Göttingen and Munich, defended a thesis project based on the studies on depression at Max Planck Institute of Psychiatry, Munich and obtained her academic degree as the Doctor of Medicine in 1972. Her major specializations are the following: Family Medicine, Psychosomatic Medicine, Psychotherapy, Hypnosis, Catathymic Imaginative Therapy, Supervision, Balint group leader. She has been working in private practice in Family Medicine (1973 to 1991) and in Medical Psychotherapy and Psychosomatics from 1986 until today.

Dr. Heide Otten has a comprehensive background in Balint work worldwide as:

- Balint group member since 1979

- Balint group leader since 1988, leading Balint groups for GPs, for gynecologists, for psychiatrists, mixed groups, for students, for teachers; groups meeting regularly, groups at weekend workshops, in Congresses, in different countries, for Psychosomatic Basic Training

- Facilitator of Balint group Leaders' Seminars, Leaders' Training and Supervision since 1995

- General Secretary of the German Balint Society 1991 to 2013

- President of the International Balint Federation (IBF) 2001 to 2007

- Member and present Vice president of the Foundation for Psychosomatic and Social Medicine „Ascona Foundation", which awards the Ascona Balint Student Prize

- Member of the IBF Task force group for development of Balint Leaders' Training 2009 to 2015

- Leader of Balint groups and Leaders' Seminars in Balint Congresses in several IBF member countries.

Dr. Heide Otten has been integrating Sculpture into Balint work and has been promoting the development of Balint movement in China and Russia.

Due to a wide spectrum of professional interests, knowledge and skills, Dr. Heide Otten also became known as:

- Teacher in Training for nurses 1972 to 1976

- Academic Teacher at the Medical School of Hannover 1999 to 2003

- Member of the board for Psychotherapeutic training and conferences in Lübeck, Lindau and Langeoog 1992 to 2014

- Team supervisor in Psychiatric Clinics and in a Haemato-oncological Ward.

Family: 3 children (born 1969, 1973, 1978), all three medical doctors (specialized in facial surgery, orthopedics and pediatrics); married to medical doctors (specialized as GP, in internal medicine and in pediatrics). Two grandsons, three granddaughters.

TABLE OF CONTENTS

1. Who was Michael Balint?

Michael Balint was born in Budapest on December 3rd, 1896. His father was a medical doctor and worked as a GP in Budapest. As well as studying medicine, Michael was interested in medical science and in psychoanalysis, which was represented and developed by Sigmund Freud (1856-1939) and Josef Breuer (1842-1925) in Vienna. Balint read Freud's books and followed his ideas. Early on he was interested in psychosomatic diseases and thought about the importance of psychological understanding in being a doctor. His idea was to sensitize GPs to the understanding, that besides the physical causes of a disease, there are psychic influences which play an important role. He discussed these matters with colleagues in London in a group, which he called „Training cum Research Group in Relationship".

He had developed the idea of the practitioner's influence on the patient and his illness during his research on drugs in Warburg's Biochemical Institute in Berlin, where he scientifically examined the effects and side effects of drugs. His idea was that the medical doctor as a person has effects and unwanted side effects on the patient, which is just like a drug. The way the doctor talks to the patient and the way he offers medication has an effect on the patient's recovery. This is what he wanted to explore with his GP groups. He reported his findings in his book „The doctor, his patient and the illness" (Balint 1957).

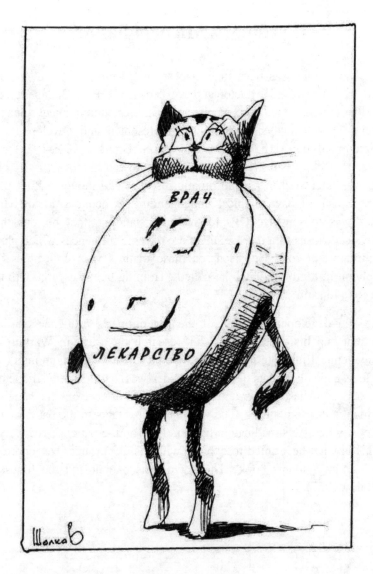

...doctor as a drug...

2. What is a Balint group?

Michael Balint (1896-1970) started this kind of group work with GPs in London after the Second World War. War-traumatized patients appeared in GPs' practices with psychosomatic reactions. It was difficult for the doctors to understand and manage these symptoms. They asked Balint to train them. So Balint thought of training the group participants in psychosomatic thinking and at the same time discover the effects of the „doctor drug": the influence of the doctor-patient relationship on diagnosis and treatment.

Today, Balint groups are used for training and to better understand the difficulties in professional relationships of the helping professions. This understanding is a relief for the helpers, avoids burn out and improves outcomes for patients and clients.

Nowadays, the officially formulated goal of the participation in Balint groups is:

- improvement in introspection;
- to recognize the importance of the helper-patient relationship;
- to improve the ability to cope with emotions;
- improvement in the perception of the influence of ways of communication;
- as Balint put it: to get to know about the effects and unwanted side effects of the doctor-patient interaction.

A „classical" Balint group

In a classical Balint group 8 to 12 members sit in a circle with one or two leaders. One of the members presents a case. He tells the story of one of his patients/clients, asking for help to understand what is going on in this professional relationship. The presenter does not use any notes and speaks freely. It is as interesting to notice what he mentions as what he neglects to tell. Factual clarifying questions can be asked after his presentation. He is not interrupted while telling the story. That gives one an impression of the presenter's mood and emotions. It may be that no question is asked, or a lot of questions are asked and seem to be important. This could already be part of the parallel process. We will come back to this later. After this part of the process the leader asks the presenter to move back a little and listen to the group members for a while without intervening. This gives him the opportunity to attend to the feedback he gets from telling his story and to his own emotions. If he stays in the group work all the time, he might feel obliged to correct or to answer more questions or to defend himself or the patient. In the pushback he is more in the situation of the patient, who does not participate in the doctor's thoughts and feelings. This can be another aspect of the parallel process. In this way, the presenter is able to be aware of the emotions evoked and expressed in the group by his telling of the story. When he is asked back into the circle he may express his feelings or add something which came to his mind and might be very important. The leader may ask him to lean back and listen again. The group now works with the new information. Before the group closes the presenter is asked back to again express his thoughts, changes and emotions.

This is an analytical group setting. The participants work with free associations, phantasies, pictures, ideas, thoughts. Balint invited the group members to „think fresh" and **„have the courage of your own stupidity"**, meaning not to use notes or study and refer to literature, but: „each of us using what he has" (Balint 1957). The presenter can choose which comment is useful to him. Sometimes he remembers only a statement when he next meets the patient and then scales fall from his eyes.

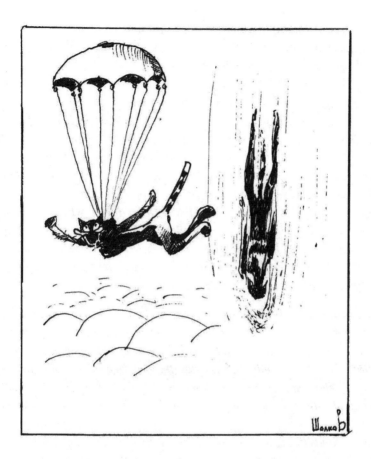

...*have the courage of your own stupidity...*

Example 1. *A young GP presents a 54 years old female patient. At her first visit in the GP's practice the patient was accompanied by her 34 years old son. She could hardly walk, suffering from severe abdominal pain. After careful inspection and questioning the doctor decides to send her to a gynecologist for further investigations. The result was cervical carcinoma. Already the patient's mother had died of cervical carcinoma. Treatment in the clinic followed, but the patient declines chemotherapy and radiation after a short period and* *goes home. The GP tries to convince her to go on with the treatment and the patient refuses. Finally the GP does home visits to care for the patient and the family. The patient has 8 children and the youngest daughter is 13 years old. The GP organizes help and psychological assistance. One of the daughters had been married in Pakistan, been divorced and had come back leaving her 4 children behind. She was depressed and had made a suicidal attempt. The family doctor – our presenter – organizes psychological support for her as well. The patient looks at a hospice and decides to go there. She asks the presenter to accompany her until the end and the doctor agrees. But the doctor feels mad with the patient: why did she not come earlier for treatment, she could have done better, this carcinoma could have been treated successfully. Why did the patient not care better for herself? She had always been present for her family; 8 children: an exhausting job ....*

The group agrees with the presenter in the first place. Then a group member emphasizes how much she admires the service the presenter gave to this patient and her family, what an engagement, what an effort. How long could she manage to work like this? Does she care for all her patients in the same way? Isn't that far too much? Suddenly the presenter has tears in her eyes. She is overwhelmed that the group appreciates her work. At the same time she understands that she behaves almost like this mother with her 8 children: she cares for all the others a lot, but not enough for herself. She is sad for the patient that she did not notice this fact in time and thankful that her eyes were opened by the group about her own behaviour and future engagement.

The Balint group does not work to find a solution. The group gives ideas, examples, different perspectives and new insights into the emotions of the presenter and the patient. That is what the presenter takes home. Unconscious contents of the relationship become conscious.

Balint groups with additional elements

Since Balint formed his first group with GPs in London the development of psychotherapy and its tools have changed and developed. Besides Freud's „talking cure" we use a lot of creative elements as techniques in single or group psychotherapeutic treatments: role-play, psychodrama, sculpturing and imagination. These creative elements help to better identify emotions to make the unconscious conscious.

In **role-play** one plays or replays a situation and a dialogue, which has taken place or could take place during the consultation. When the presenter slips into the patient's shoes, he feels the potency of the words, which he himself had used or might use in the real situation. Different group members may role-play and one can feel the nuances and differences. This way one becomes aware of what transference and counter transference mean. Changing roles helps to increase understanding and to develop empathy.

Example 2. This example may show how role-play can help one better understand the situation of a doctor-patient-interaction: Jenny, a young GP felt helpless and incompetent handling a 76 years old non-compliant patient. He suffered from severe back pain, especially in his neck. He used to drop in without an appointment when he felt he needed something but missed appointments at other times and did not consult the specialists as agreed with the GP. He always brought his wife with him and she had dementia. He claimed that he could not leave her at home alone. That was also his excuse for not having further investigations.

The group expressed sympathy with the doctor, who wanted to help but could not. They felt the frustration, the helplessness and the anger. One group member identified with the patient and talked about his burden, his loneliness and the sadness. Getting old is not easy, and nowadays we do not live in big families any more, where you could distribute tasks and find support. Almost everybody knew patients like this.

The presenter listened carefully. When she moved back into the group, she said she was thankful for the understanding and loyalty shown to her. But she still felt powerless. She would prefer to send him to a specialist clinic to offer some rest for him, but she was sure that he would not accept that and then she would be angry with him.

The leader offered a role-play. Jenny played the patient, a female psychiatrist in the group played Jenny's role, the GP.

The patient entered the room, bent, stiff neck, pain-distorted face, sat down and complained. The doctor reacted very calmly, listened and said: „I understand" – „I see" – „That is a difficult situation" .... „You really worked a lot during your life, that was hard work as a mason. You deserve a rest." .... „There are clinics which would take both of you, you and your wife. She may need some treatment for her dementia, too. And you in the meantime could get really effective pain relief. The clinic takes good care of both of you." Patient: „Ok, I will think about it. — But can you do something against my pain now?" – „Yes, let's go to the desk for a prescription."...

Jenny was overwhelmed. She had felt the tension in her body and the pain, especially in her neck. She felt the burden on her shoulders bodily. And she was surprised how good it felt when the doctor was just listening, with empathy, not trying to convince her. The GP had an offer to make, nothing more, nor less — no pressure, just something to think about. She was not ashamed, had no resistance against the GP's suggestion. Somebody cared. It was a warm feeling.

„ I am very much looking forward to the next consultation now. The patient has an appointment next Friday. I hope he will be there!"

Role-play makes it easier and even more effective to change the perspective.

Psychodrama is extended role-play, developed by Moreno. Balint work and Moreno's idea of being creative by improvising fit well together. Moreno's concept of spontaneity explains the Balint group dynamics as well: an old situation." (Moreno 1974). „Precondition for change in relationships is the growth in the premier quality to act in a way, which is necessary breaking up fixations.... the spontaneous person acts as if he was a beginner. Every moment is new" (Krüger 1997). This matches Balint's invitation „to **think fresh"**.

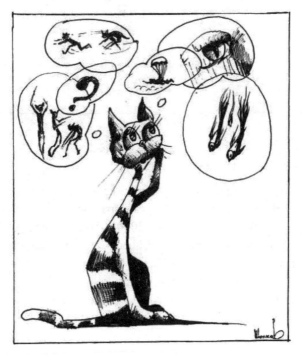

...think fresh...

He expects the group members to engage in the situation, to focus on the feelings of the moment, and to fully concentrate on the story presented.

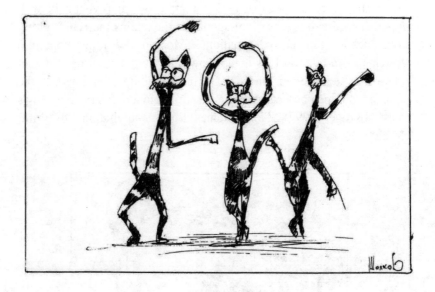

...sculpture...

Creating a **sculpture** is a systemic approach. The method was developed in family therapy by Virginia Satir (1916-1988) in the 1970s. Thea Schönfelder (1925-2010) demonstrated the method impressingly in the 1980s in Lübeck at the Northern German Psychotherapy week. The group members are representing the "figures" involved in the problematic relationship as part of the sculpture, the presenter is given the chance to look at his problem and himself being represented by somebody else, too, from a distance. This distance can help him to see more clearly, discover blind spots and gain new impressions; the quality of affect and emotion will change. Body language is an effective ingredient.

Imagination helps us to find pictures for the presented problems instead of rationalizing. We tend to „think" about the problem instead of feeling, what this relationship might be like. The result could be to offer solutions before having really understood what is going on between the protagonists. Rationalization is a defence. The group sometimes tends to share the defence with the presenter. Imagination helps us to get new ideas and new insights.

Example 3. *Christiane is a family practitioner working in a rural area. As usual in the countryside she sees patients of all ages. A 16 years old girl comes, together with her mother, comes to see Christiane. The girl demands two transfers to specialists in a very disrespectful manner. Christiane asks what she wants from the referrals and the girl answers cheekily. Finally she unwillingly shows the doctor a little dry spot on her skin, which really does not need examination by a dermatologist. Christiane gives her a prescription. She offers the girl an explanation for her other problem: the girl had self-diagnosed Raynaud phenomenon – her fingers sometimes turned white – and and she had researched it on the internet. Now she wanted a specialist examination. Christiane explained that this was not appropriate and made another appointment for a week later. The girl came back with her mother and said the cream did not help. Nevertheless her skin was better. The girl's mother did not say a thing. Christiane felt hurt, humiliated and angry. „If it was my daughter I would have put her on the spot. She has to respect a grown up, a doctor, and not behave like that. She should study Knigge. Spoiled girl! Bad upbringing!"*

The group members fully agreed. Oh, those adolescents from today – how badly they behave. A problem everywhere, in school, in the public .... Most of the remarks started „I think ..." or „ I would... "

The leader asks the group members to pause for a short while, just close their eyes and let their imagination float. Six minutes later the leader asks the participants to take a deep breathe, open the eyes and and come back to talk about their images: – there was a little princess in a pink dress, a 3 years old stomping with the foot, crying, nobody comes, she cries louder, mother gives her a sweet and leaves..., – a stylish teenage girl at a party, trying to appear cool, arrogant, snobbish, hiding her uncertainty, her frustration and disgust, lonely..... – a girl in front of her big mirror, looking at her face, at her body, at her skin, not satisfied with what she sees, while her mother exclaims: „You look so pretty!" it sounds feigned „You are a liar, you do not really look at me!"

...a mother with raised index finger: „Behave!" She takes a walk with two little well dressed kids on her right and left hand.... – a duck family crossing the street, mother first, three little ducks following in a row...

The atmosphere in the group had changed with the imagination part. What was the real problem for the girl? What did she really want to express? Why did she consult the GP? Why did she bring her mother? And what was the doctor's frustration? Christiane's anger vanished. She was surprised that she had almost forgotten that the mother was in the room. Now she understood that the mother had been very important, that she was angry at her, competing with her, that this mother had done such a bad job, bringing up this girl, that she did not limit her daughter, did not teach her appropriately. And now she realized that under the arrogance and cheeky appearance of the youngster there was an unhappy, uncertain, unsatisfied child, whose real needs were hidden, not experienced, not seen. „As her GP, I would like to get to know this girl better" was Christianes closing remark.

Imagination helped to find a way to the emotional level, to interrupt a moral and political discussion, to leave predudices behind and look under the surface, to get to the emotions beneath the arrogance and disrespectful manner. And the presenter understood that she was in competition with the mother, thought of educating her better than her mother did, instead of analyzing the presentation of the girl's symptoms as a request to really look at her.

Some Balintians are skeptical and ask: "Is this still Balint work?" Balint was especially interested in new therapeutic techniques in his time, eg. the focal therapy. Adding new techniques to his „training cum research groups" might have evoked his interest.

To use these additional elements in Balint work requires Balint group leaders to have special knowledge. We will come back to that later.

The „Fishbowl" group

When Michael Balint was invited for a weekend workshop to Sils Maria in Switzerland he was surprised by the great number of participants. He was used to working with a small group with up to 10 group members. Now he found 30 colleagues waiting for him. They all wanted to experience a group with him as leader. He had to find a solution. And this was what we call the „Fishbowl" today. The working group of 8 to 12 members is sitting in the center surrounded by the other participants. As far as I know, in Balint's setting they were just watching the process. We use fishbowl these days as demonstration groups in congresses etc.

Nowadays we are also aware of more possibilities; the outer circle can add to the group process. These participants listen to the story from a greater distance. Different emotions, associations and phantasies may be evoked in them. When they listen to the discussion of the group members in the inner circle they might feel different. So during the group process the leaders can use these circumstances and give the outer circle the chance to express their thoughts, feelings, phantasies, enriching the group work of the inner circle.

Example 4. A group at a Balint weekend-workshop is created by participants volunteering to sit in the inner circle. This time it is 8 group members, 24 more sitting around in an outer circle. The group consists of GPs, Psychiatrists, Gynecologists and one pediatrician. The group leader explains that the inner group will work as a usual

Balint group. The outer circle will have to listen. Maybe he would invite the outer circle to give their votes and express their impressions when he thinks it might be helpful for the inner group.

A GP presents a case. He is a family doctor in his village where he grew up. His father had worked in this practice before him. He knows most of the people – now his patients – from former times. Sometimes this makes his work and his doctor-patient-relationships difficult. He wants to talk about a patient, who has been his schoolmate and is now his neighbour. Their wives and children are good friends. Last year this man developed a bipolar disorder. He was hospitalized for 3 months, then came back and asked his friend to take care of him. Everything went fine until he stopped his medication. Very soon he became manic. He then tried to get close to the GP's wife. She defended herself against him and he became very angry. In this situation he dragged her to the balcony and was about to push her down. The doctor was very upset; on one hand he is furious about this action, on the other hand he does not want to leave his friend alone in the difficult situation. He considers his severe illness. He feels helpless, the situation hopeless.

The group takes up the doctor's anger in the first place, then his worries and helplessness. Some of the female participants identify with his wife. She has a hard time and, of course, should be certain about her husband's ability to protect her. Others understand his ambivalence. On top of it all, the families are close, not only as neighbors. After a while the group work seems to go in a circle. When the leader gets aware of this, he decides to ask the outer circle for their impressions. The emotions outside the group seemed to be far less intense. They acknowledge the ambivalence, the anger, the fears, but they have a more distant and professional view of the situation. They talk about the role confusion: being friend, family doctor, GP, Psychiatrist, social worker .... all at the same time. That is too much. What a burden. They are looking for more shoulders to put the weight on.

The inner group is relieved. Now they are able to phantasize about a different setting. And the presenter is relieved, too. He now feels free to engage other professionals; he is ready to ask his GP colleague to take care of the family. He decided to serve as a good friend, not more and not less.

The **fishbowl** offers this opportunity to get input from a greater distance. Maybe the small group would have come to this point in itself later. The leader could have made a corresponding intervention. But why not use the observations from the outside?

„Fishbowl" groups are usually offered in Congresses and weekend workshops with more than one small group registered.

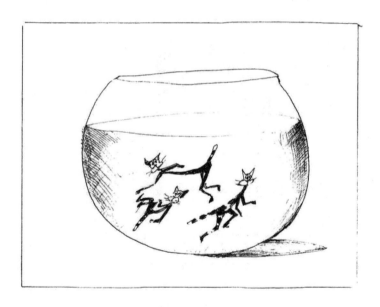

...*fishbowl*...

The Leaders' Seminar

The „fishbowl" setting is also used in the leaders' seminars. Ideally 15 participants form a group for the leaders' training. We will come to the requirements to enter the **leaders' training** later.

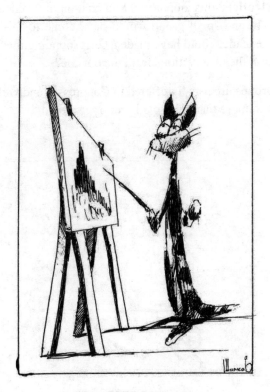

...leaders' training...

In the Leaders' Seminars everybody has the opportunity to experience the different positions – participant, presenter, leader or co-leader, observer outside the group – allowing understanding of what is going on in a Balint group. During training one has to be in these different positions. In this way one finds out about group dynamics, group process, parallel process and the influence the leaders' interventions and behavior have on the group work, the group members and the outcomes for the presenter.

As a **group member**: What was your experience? Did the leaders take good care of you? Did they protect you? Did they notice when you wanted to say something and did not get the opportunity? Were you able to speak freely, express your emotions, „think fresh" or say something „dumb" — as Balint expressed it — or have the „courage of your own stupidity"?

It is important to make use of free associations, not filtered by reasoning or doubts. All contributions are like flowers — the presenter may take this bunch of flowers home, keep the smell in his mind. It will pop up when he meets the patient again.

And did the leaders respect what you said? Did they value your thoughts?

The leader has an influence on ranking ideas and contributions. When he stresses it or repeats what a member has said, it stays more in mind.

And if discomfort is expressed, were the leaders able to accept it or maybe explain it afterwards as part of the case dynamics? If he does, every member feels free even to express anger, disgust, envy – all the emotions we think we should not have as a professional.

As a **presenter**: What was that like? Did you feel safe in the group; especially when the leaders asked you to push back and just listen while the group worked on your patient relationship? It takes a lot of trust to present a story and for a while not to have any influence on the group process. It is important that the leaders keep contact with the presenter, not abandon him in **the pushback position** and ask him back when they feel the need to do so. The leaders have to react when group members attack or devalue the presenter's work. Do you remember how they supported ideas and diminished others? A very interesting task of the leaders is to see the parallel process and make it visible for the group. We will come back to this important issue later.

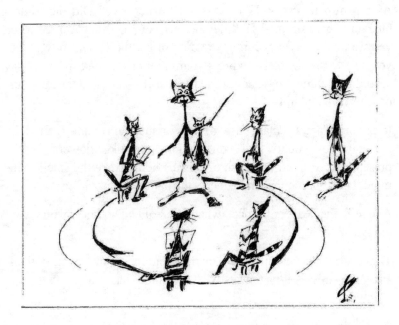

...pushback position...

An **observer** participates in the Balint group process, but sits outside the group watching what happens in the group.

In this position one follows the group dynamics. One watches what the leaders' interventions create. One can sometimes guess the leader's hypotheses about the relationship, when he tries to convince the group or underlines certain remarks and does not pay attention to others. Or one notices that the leader is open to different ideas and that he is able to take new perspectives into account.

One watches the two leaders, how they work together, whether they distribute their tasks, whether they are in competition or support each other's position. They play different roles in the process; they are objects of transference and countertransference. Did they notice this and how did they deal with it?

As one of the **leaders**: Did you sense uncertainty in yourself? What was it like to be in this position for the first time? Could you rely on your co-leader? It is not easy to always pay attention to the presenter, to the group members, to the group process, to the parallel process and to your own emotions.

It sounds quite exhausting to be in the position of group leader. It is a challenge. Fortunately there are some aspects that provide relief. The good thing is that as a leader one has time to reflect while the group is working.

We usually take 90 minutes for the group process, dealing with one relationship. That gives the possibility to listen carefully and in a relaxed way, to the presenter's story and to the group's comments. And while listening, one can reflect on one's own emotions, on countertransference, on the story and on the group process.

When the group members ask, for example, their clarifying questions, the leaders notice what is asked and what is not asked. Why did nobody want to know whether the patient had a family? Why did nobody ask about his social life, about his sexuality, about his job? You keep it in mind and maybe come back to it later if it is not mentioned by one of the group members. Maybe it has a meaning.

While the group starts working one can, as a leader, focus on one's own emotions for a moment and find out about one's own hypotheses concerning the relationship. At the same time one listens to the opinions and watches the presenter's reactions.

If the story provokes a strong emotion in you as a leader, you are lucky to have a Co-leader, who observed it and relieves you of following the group process until you come back to a leading position.

As leader one **oscillates between the emotional and the meta position**. This way one is connected with oneself, one's own emotions, thoughts, memories, experiences, transference and countertransference, with one's co-leader, with the presenter, with the group and with the case.

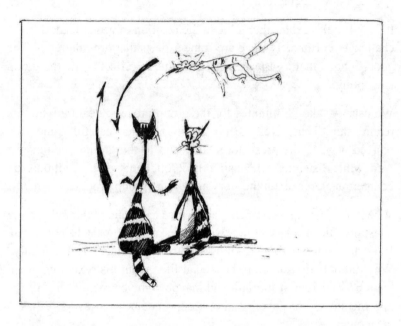

…oscillate between the emotional and the meta position…

Like in Psychotherapy our transference and countertransference, our empathy and emotional reactions are the instruments we work with as a Balint group leader. The doctor „must learn to use himself as skillfully as the surgeon uses his knife, the physician his stethoscope, the radiologist his lamps" (Balint 1957) — and so must the Balint group leader. That is why **self experience training** is demanded before starting the Leader's Training.

We are working with a group. That is why knowledge about **group dynamics** is necessary.The setting in a Balint group is what makes it effective and special and distinguish it from other group settings. Group dynamics is most important and it often mirrors the case. That is what we use as an important instrument in Balint group work.

In the Leaders' Training sessions we usually take 45 minutes for the group work and the other 45 minutes to discuss the group process from all the different positions: How did the group members feel? What did the observers observe? Did the presenter feel safe and what did he get out of the process? What was the leaders' goal? Did they have a hypothesis about the difficulties in the doctor-patient-relationship? Were they open to new aspects? Did they feel well and certain in their roles? Did the leader mention the parallel process? What was the leaders' influence on the group process? And what supported the outcomes for the presenter?

3. What a Balint group is not

A case discussion group

When we think of a Balint group, we have in mind that it needs phantasy, free associations, the expression of emotions, the focus on the doctor-patient-relationship. In a case discussion group, we rationally focus on diagnosis and treatment in the first place. We want to know all the facts about the physical examination, blood tests, x-rays, MRIs etc. In a psychiatric case we, of course, are looking at transference and countertransference, also as a diagnostic tool. The treatment is discussed based on all diagnostic findings. We use the patient's medical record, our rationality and emotions.

A therapy group

The leader of a therapy group is the specialist and the group members are patients. The leader uses the group dynamics, transference and countertransference to treat the patients in the group. Defended emotions and energies become visible in the group and are used for understanding and recovery. The group members get a social training interacting with each other. They get open feedback on their behavior. They learn to cope with conflicts and solve them, to deal with their own aggression, envy etc and that of others. The social competence of the group members grows. The relationships within the group are focused upon. New experiences in a protected environment are offered.

Supervision

Supervision is offered in different settings.

There is team supervision in departments to improve the atmosphere and the working process. The group and the supervisor set goals to first find out what is not going well and then find solutions together. The content of these discussions is the practical work, the different roles in the team and the dynamic of the interaction.

A case supervision group focusses on the dynamics between the team and the patient/client/student. This comes close to Balint work. The relationship between the professional and his client is important. Transference and countertransference are taken into account. The difference is that one looks for a solution and works with facts and organizational problems and tries to solve them.

Supervision in training for helping professions, e.g. for psychiatrists and psychotherapists, focusses on diagnosis and therapy. It is obligatory for trainees. It is meant to be guidance of the therapeutic activities of the doctor in training by an experienced colleague during the whole therapeutic treatment of the patient. One does not take more than four trainees in a supervision group. The doctors in training learn more about the patients. They discuss the psychotherapeutic techniques and learn from each other. It is a case discussion. Group dynamics is not the essential tool as in Balint work.

Supervision has a teaching aspect, whereas Balint work is a stimulus to be open to new insights and changes of perspective.

A self-experience group

During your training to become a psychotherapist you have to join a self-experience group. There you learn a lot about your own psychodynamics, emotions, motives, actions and reactions, your transference and countertransference. All these are tools, which you need in your profession. Balint said you have to be able to use these tools as well as a surgeon uses his knife. Similar to the therapy group, the group member and his behavior is in the focus. To get to know about your own defended emotions and energies is most important before you treat patients. You learn to switch roles with other people, change perspectives. This way you learn to better understand yourself and the patient.

There is always self-experience in Balint group work, too. When you get the group's feedback on your relationship with the patient, you learn a lot about yourself. You get aware of your own motives and difficulties when you talk about your relationship with a patient. This is not the only focus. It may well be a stimulus to reflect more about one's self. The self-experience group would look for the roots of your emotional reactions and behaviour, at your family of origin, your life situation, your deep emotions, e.g. concerning your partnership. In a Balint group that stays unsaid and unasked.

For a Balint group leader it is indispensable to have self-awareness. When he is sitting in the group, he has to oscillate between emotions and the meta position. To be able to do so, he has to be aware of his own emotions and reactions, his own transference and countertransference, and he has to be able to differentiate and deal with these. Acting them out would destroy the group work.

The group-work has elements of a self experience-process, not only for the presenter but for all group members. They all get to know more about themselves without talking about their privacy. The focus is not the personality of the doctor and his private life but the doctor-patient-relationship and the understanding of the patient's signals and symptoms and the doctor's unconscious answers.

Analyzing the doctor-patient-relationship means both: seeing the patient's conflicts, needs, suffering, illness and the doctor's conscious and unconscious reactions.

4. What is the leader's position in a Balint group?

My most important teacher in this field was Werner Stucke, and he used to say: „As a Balint group leader you can do everything, nothing is wrong, you just have to be aware of what you are doing". I would like to add: „and you have to be aware of your own attitudes towards the presenter, the case, the group members etc. and what your interventions create..."

On the one hand, the leader is part of the group process. He is listening to the case presentation just like the group members. He has his own thoughts, feelings, his hypotheses about the doctor, the patient and their relationship. At the same time, he is directing the group process, watching the reactions of the group members and intervening. He is thinking about how to structure the process with a balance of enabling, giving room, structuring and limiting – not too much, not too little. For example, considering when to stop the presentation by the presenter. Are questions wanted and fruitful, or is it better to ask the group for their emotions and reactions right away? How many questions? If there are many questions, should the leader stop it and how? Or should he let it go and remark „what does this mean to ask a lot of questions?" When to bring a new idea in or summarize or give a comment on the discussion that is going on.

The leader's decisions influence the group process. What is the outcome? And does this have anything to do with the case, with the doctor-patient-relationship? Are we working for the presenter? Is he still the focus? Should he be taken out or brought back in?

While listening to the group the leader makes all his decisions consciously. And he watches the reactions in the group with his **free-floating attention**.

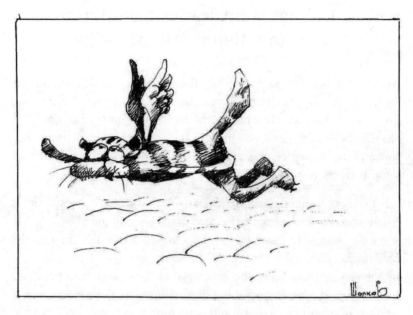

...free-floating attention...

Let us suggest that the leader has a strong hypothesis and tries to bring the group to follow it. What can happen? Maybe they follow him, or maybe there is resistance. If he does not notice and stays in the resistance with the group, the discussion will be narrow, reluctant, going in a circle. If he does notice, after a while, that he is going in a different direction from where the group is going, he can either make a remark about it, trying to convince the group, or he can follow the thoughts and expressions of the group members. He may then change his hypothesis and get new ideas. He follows the group discussion witn an open mind with free gliding attention.

He keeps an eye on the presenter, on his safety, his reactions, his need to come back into the group discussion and on the main subject: the doctor-patient-relationship.

Example 5. *A young GP presents a case. He has been working in his father's private practice for half a year. His father wants to retreat step by step with our colleague taking over more responsibility. There is an old couple he has to care for. His father told him: „Watch out. Especially, she is not easy to handle. Until 15 years ago she was a nurse in our community. She is a little bit bossy." When the young doctor makes his first home visit, he can feel what his father tried to tell him. He talks to the husband, but always gets an answer from his wife. She does not want the doctor to examine him, she just wants him to give a prescription and leave. He is unhappy about the situation, because he saw things going wrong. For example, the former nurse gave emergency medication to her husband, which made the situation worse. He tried very carefully to explain, but she would not listen. She emphasises that she has a lot of medical experience while he is far too young to know. She does not take him and his advice seriously. He tries again during two subsequent house calls. Then he gives up and asks her to look for another doctor. He is relieved on one side but unhappy on the other. And he does not understand why he is unhappy. He has lots of patients, more than enough to care about, nice ones who accept his advice.*

The hypothesis of the group leader may be: the doctor is afraid of his father's judgement. He feels, that he failed. He did not manage to get along with the difficult patient. With this hypothesis in mind, he stresses all statements in the group, which follow his direction. The group leader may state: „Well, it is not easy to succeed his father." And the group will phantasize about this subject. Hopefully a group member or the co-leader (if there is one) leads the attention back to the two patients. „What about the old man. I pity him. He did not have the chance to relate to the doctor. Maybe he likes him." That would be an important new perspective.

If the group leader sticks to his hypothesis he would probably come back to it, either by giving this thought little chance to develop („If he really liked him, would he then have dropped him?"), or by asking something about the structure of the practice ("What about losing or abandoning patients? Might this be a subject for the presenter's father?")

A leader who is open to new ideas and perspectives would follow this trace. "Ok. You felt that he liked the old man. How would our presenter feel about him now?" Someone else could look at the old nurse. Is she just arrogant? Is she anxious? Does she want control? What experience has she gained with doctors during her professional life?

The leader with his strong hypothesis may ask: "Or is she just as suspicious towards the young doctor as his father is of him? Does the father really trust him? Is he sure that he can rely on his son and entrust his patients to him." The leader who is open-minded might find this aspect interesting and support it: "That is a good question. Did she really mistrust the young doctor? Maybe she just wanted to express her anxiety and doubts. Maybe she looked for a fatherly, certain doctor, who calmed her down and assured her of the right tools for emergency situations."

Balint work does not look for solutions. The group offers phantasies, emotions, associations and thoughts to the presenter like a bunch of flowers. The presenter then decides what is important for him, what enlightens his blind spots, what gives him new ideas; this may even be later after the group work, maybe when he meets the patient again. The leader stimulates and collects all these suggestions from the group members. In our case he would be open to all aspects: the presenter's relationship to his father, to the patient, to the patient's wife, his uncertainty, his ideal, his boundaries etc.

Listening to the presenter's story, everybody in the group develops a quick hypothesis. You can feel it when the group members give their first impression. "Think fresh" was Michael Balint's invitation. All contributions are precious and reflect unconscious and conscious inputs of the presenter. The leader in his meta position has to differentiate his own spontaneous hypothesis from the enriching comments in the group.

Whenever he has a co-leader, he keeps in contact with him. Having two leaders in the group is supposed to be a relief. They can divide up all the important responsibilities and duties.The most important thing is that both oscillate from listening attentively to the **meta position**, watching what is going on and how they both influence the process. And that is what training people consists of in the leaders' workshops.

It is not a question of right and wrong, good or bad. It is the question of **self recognition** and **awareness**.

The tasks the leader has learned as a group member, such as listening patiently and carefully to the contributions of the others, being respectful, feeling safe enough to fantasize and „think fresh" are needed for leading a group himself.

The different experiences of being a member of a group, leading or co-leading under supervision and observing the group work from the outside are important ingredients of the training and learning process.

The analysis of the group process, the leader's influence on the group work and the atmosphere in the group are done in the second half of the leaders' training session. A well-trained leader has these in mind while leading the group and making his interventions.

To lead a Balint group can be looked at as a technique, which only works well with self awareness.

Guido Flatten found in his investigation that the group members experience and describe the presence and actions of the leaders as the most important influence on their work.

And Balint wrote: „*Perhaps the most important factor is the behavior of the leader of the group. It is hardly an exaggeration to say that if he finds the right attitude he will teach more by his example than by everything else combined. After all, the technique we advocate is based on exactly the same sort of listening that we expect the doctors to learn and then to practice with their patients. By allowing everybody to be themselves, to have their say in their own way and in their own time, by watching for proper cues – that is, speaking only when something is really expected from him and making his point in a form which, instead of prescribing the right way, opens up possibilities for the doctors to discover by themselves some right way of dealing with the patient's problems – the leader can demonstrate in the ‚here and now' situation what he wants to teach.*

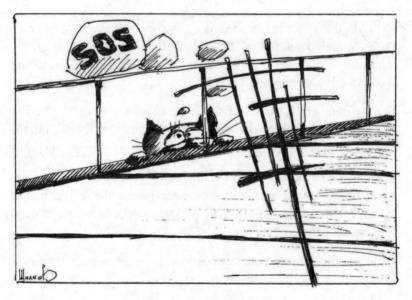

...*when something went wrong...*

Obviously no-one can live up to these exacting standards. Fortunately there is no need for perfection. The group leader may make mistakes – in fact he often does – without causing much harm if he can accept criticism in the same or even somewhat sharper terms than he expects his group to accept." (Balint 1957).

Balint points out that the leader is a model. The way he deals with statements in the group, the way he listens and gives room to new ideas and acknowledges them is a model for the interaction in the group and in the doctor-patient interaction. And just like the participant seeking for help in his Balint group, the leader may look for help from the co-leader when he feels **something went wrong**.

Ethical assumptions and limitations

The most important message the leader gives is to respect each other and to acknowledge what group members say. There may be people from different cultures, another backgrounds with different religious or world views. The patients which are presented may seem strange, their behavior incorrect, their demands too much. Respect is most important. And the question „why" is always in the air. Can we understand what is going on?

Of course there are limits to understanding and accepting. „To think fresh" does not mean to hurt, to destroy or to attack. It is often a tightrope walk for the leader to distinguish between remarks that bring the reflection forward and comments that are too much, not helpful, or only aggressive. Most important is cognition of the parallel process. Personal attacks from one group member to another cross the borderline. The leader has to make it visible and stop it. Safety in the group is most important.

In Balint groups it is not a question of right or wrong, either/or, it is the „as well as". It is important to accept contradictory thoughts and ideas and ambivalence. The success of a Balint group depends on the honesty, openness, respect and mutual support of group members. **Confidentiality** is most important. The longer the group works together the more the group cohesion and reliance grows.

Safety in the group for the presenter, for the group members

The leaders' responsibility is to keep the balance between giving room and structuring.

The group work is rich and fruitful when group members feel free to express their thoughts, phantasies and feelings in a safe atmosphere. How can the leader establish such an atmosphere? Alert, concentrated, positive, friendly, certain, strict, clear, setting boundaries – these are characteristics of a group leader, who guarantees safety and a creative atmosphere in the group. Cheeky thoughts are allowed, laughter is ok, as long as it does not hurt. Limiting these expressions does not mean to cut them off, but name them. The leader can try to give an interpretation. He can pose a question like „Why is laughter coming up at that point? Do we avoid another emotion?" „What sort of laughter is it? Is it shameful, aggressive or devaluing laughter?" The leader has to always keep an eye on the presenter, especially when he is in the pushback position. He can get the presenter back anytime and ask for his reactions.

Confidentiality

Before the group starts working the leader outlines the group rules. He reminds group members to be on time and not to leave before the group finishes. If somebody needs to leave the room, he has to signal to indicate what is going on. Confidentiality is essential. Everybody in the group has to be sure that his comments or his story as a presenter does not leave the room. This is always important and especially in clinics, where the participants know each other well. They work together, eat together, they have leisure time together. It is essential fort he group to accept, that they do not go on to discuss what happened in the group or talk about it with others. If the participants are not sure about confidentiality nobody would want to present a case and the discussion would be rational and boring.

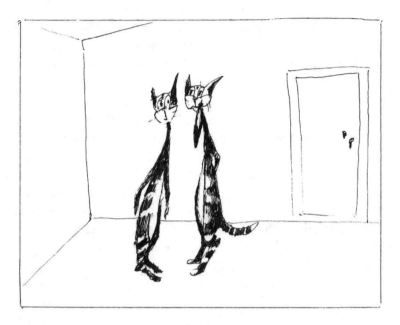

...confidentiality...

Confidentiality is the most important ingredient of Balint group work. It is one reason why we do not accept heads of the clinic together with their dependent employees in a Balint group. That would hinder a free and safe atmosphere.

To resolve conflicts

What sort of conflicts may appear in a Balint group? The leader has to differentiate between a conflict which mirrors the case and a conflict due to difficulties between members of the group. If it is a parallel process the leader has to point that out and lead the group to an understanding. In either case we know from group dynamics: „Disturbances have priority". It is one of the tasks of the leaders not to avoid them but to resolve them. And again the leader may serve as an example. How does he notice the conflict? How does he address it?

Let me give you an example. In Germany we have obligatory groups. Doctors in training have to attend Balint groups. They do not always like it. Mostly the groups are in their free time in the evening or at weekends. That leads to unwilling participation. Two members of such a group fought about details and devalued the statements of the other. The leader made his observation open and asked the group about their experience. They complained about the pressure they felt in their training, their frustration in obligatory events which they thought boring or unnecessary. A lack of free time with friends and family was everyday life. Instead of talking about patients again, they needed the opportunity to talk about their personal problems, their life situation. The leader offered this opportunity. In the next session the group was able to get back to work on the doctor-patient-relationship. The group members recognized that the Balint group focusing the doctor-patient-relationship was open to their problems. The leader set an example. Maybe the young colleagues took home that listening to a patient's problem instead of just taking a blood test and bodily examination might be a good investment of time.

How to deal with aggression

Aggression, in the first place, is an energy. We can use it for moving, for bringing things forward, for leaving dependencies. Aggression in a Balint group may appear as a confrontation, e.g. confronting the presenter with his unconscious fears, desires and needs. „Think fresh" may mean making aggression overt.

„I would hate this patient with all his demands..." – „I have an ugly thought, I would kick him out..." To know about aggressive impulses and tendencies gives a feeling of freedom and relief. Just to phantasize that you could give the person a kick maybe makes you laugh – what a relief. In this way aggressive fantasies are welcome in a Balint group.

It becomes difficult when it is not acknowledged as a welcome fantasy but instead acted out: aggression may appear as devaluation, an insult or an offense. Even an open war of words may appear in the group.

The group leader's task is to find out what it means. Is it part of the doctor-patient-relationship? Does the aggressive group mirror the case? Or does this aggressive dynamics come from other sources? One of these sources may be that it is an obligatory group and the participants are so fed up with talking about patients all the time. They would rather discuss other subjects or be with their families or friends. Another reason could be an unknown rivalry between members of the group, or unsolved conflicts from other places. The leader has to find out about it, which means to speak openly.

In this field self-experience of the leader is extremely important. Did he learn to deal with aggression? Or was it taboo in his family of origin? And has it been taboo in his profession? An aggressive doctor — unbelievable. A doctor has to be always nice, understanding and empathetic. If the leader has a similar ideal, it will be hard to accept deeper emotions, which do not fit into this ideal. If a leader learned to be afraid of aggressive emotions and seeks to appease, he will probably fail to make use of aggression in the Balint group. Instead he might provoke tendencies towards defence and inhibition of aggression resulting in a tense atmosphere within the group.

Aggression which points towards the leader himself is not easy to handle. He has to find the reason. Is it a parallel process? Does it mirror the case? Did he start a fight with the group?

Example 6. *Some members of a Balint group arrived for their meeting distressed with the news that the authorities wanted to cut their incomes using new regulations. They wanted to urgently discuss the organisational changes instead of dealing with a doctor-patient-relationship. The Balint group leader asked them to postpone this* *discussion to the coffee brake and start with Balint work right away. After some protest one of them presented a case.*

The patient was a nurse in the presenter's practice. His problem was that she wanted a lengthy sick certificate after a surgical procedure. He asked her to take his financial situation into account, saying in addition that he could not afford to pay for a replacement. The group followed his arguments and criticized the patient/clerk. The discussion about the GPs' financial situation was opened up. When the leader intervened: „I have the impression that other important aspects in this case have not been mentioned so far" he attracted the aggression of the group members, whom he had rejected before.

An experienced leader might have been able to analyze the situation together with an experienced group. „I understand that you are cross with me because I pushed through to talk about a doctor-patient-relationship. And I see, you were clever enough to come back to your desired subject: the financial changes. One to zero for you!" (smiling).

In this case it was an uncertain leader with a new compulsory group. He talked about this experience in a supervision group for Balint group leaders. Hopefully, he understood and at the next meeting was able to talk openly with the group.

5. What is the Co-leader's job?

It is of benefit to work in a Balint group with two leaders. You may divide the tasks, which, as we learned, are multiple. The two leaders sit in the group opposite each other, so they have different perspectives. One of them can watch the presenter and his reactions and take good care of him. When the presenter is in the pushback situation it is necessary to notice when he needs to come back.

One of the leaders usually conducts the process, the other one observes it. If the story provokes strong emotions in one of the leaders, you are lucky to have a Co-leader, who notices and relieves the partner by following the group process until the other one comes back to his leading position.

It is important for the co-leaders to be aware of their degree of cooperation. If the two co-leaders know each other well and have been working together for some time they can make use of their observations. Why are they fighting today? Is this a parallel process due to the case? Why are they competing? Are doctor and patient in competition? Does the group try to split them? What does that mean? Are they acting like parents, mothering and fathering the group or the presenter? This helps them understand the process. The group feels safe when the two leaders act openly and verbalize their positions.

Supporting the leader

The multiple tasks of the leaders can be shared. The two leaders communicate this before they start the group work. They agree about who will be responsible for the structure and give the inputs. It is not easy when the two have very different ideas of the case or of their leading styles. If one of them is used to giving a lot of room to group members, not intervening much and letting the group process go, and the other one is used to much more structure, it is wise to talk about these things beforehand and find a way through. One of them has to lead to bring the group to work. If the competition between the two working styles is not solved beforehand, the outcome will be poor. The group is paralyzed by the competition or the group is split and competing, too. Both will not give enough room for the presenter and the case. The goal of two leaders facilitating the group is to support each other in sharing the tasks, watching carefully and serving the group, primarily the presenter. An exchange of thoughts between the two leaders after the group session is a very valuable ingredient.

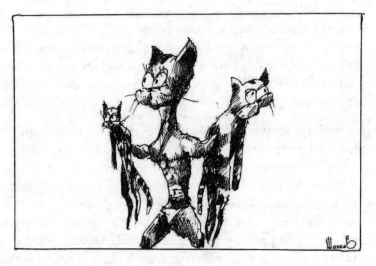

...support...

Reflecting the group process

The co-leader's job is to carefully watch the group process and offer his reflections about it to the group. One of the fascinating observations in a Balint group is the **parallel process**. I will come back to it later. Bern Carrière wrote an essay with the title: „Do the group dynamics always mirror the case?" That is a tricky and very difficult question.

Balint groups may be started in Clinics as well, where the group members have more points of contact than sitting together in a Balint group. They work together, have their meals and training together and sometimes know the same patients from different situations.

This presents a special challenge for the leaders in differentiating between team dynamics and case dynamics. It seems easier to have a group of strangers, people who never met before. But watch out. We know about transference and countertransference. There might be somebody in the group that reminds me of a colleague, my father, my sister, my aunt.... Not all the emotions in the group are evoked by the case!

Taking care of the individual group member

Both leaders concentrate on the group members. The co-leader often has more time to look around while the group leader focusses on the statements, the speakers, the presenter, the case and the parallel process. There might be a member, who is quiet, has not mentioned anything so far. The co-leader pays attention to those members especially, he watches mime, gestures, body language, and he looks for the right moment to invite this member to join the group discussion. He may ask him directly or point out that he wonders why this member keeps quiet. Sometimes these group members bring in very important aspects of the doctor-patient-relationship. „I thought, nobody would listen to me anyway" or „I have nothing to say." or „I am so angry" or „I tried to find my way into the discussion, but there was always somebody faster than I am." or „Unnecessary to say something, there is nothing to add." This individual member may represent one part of the patient. Every individual member in the group could represent one side of the patient or the presenter. It is the leaders' task to value this and make use of it. To point out that the emotions in the group mirror the case helps the individual group member. You sometimes hear e.g. „I don't know what is wrong with me, I usually do not feel that way. But here I feel abandoned, lethargic, resigned, sadistic..."

6. The Parallel Process

The story with its conflicts and emotions is reflected in the group. The presenter often gets into the position of the patient, especially in the pushback situation. He has told **his story** of his experience with a patient and confided it to the group just like the patient commits **his story** and his symptoms to the doctor. It is not rare for the patient to have doubts: Does the doctor really understand what I mean? Does he draw the right conclusions? Can he really help me?

Something similar may happen to the presenter. When he has presented the story to the group and is in the push-back position doubts may arise: Was he able to make his concerns clear? Can he trust the group, especially the leaders? What are they going to do with his request? Will he profit from the process? He may feel abandoned like the patient or well taken care of.

In the pushback situation the presenter sits outside, is excluded from the discussion for a while — just like the patient is in a way excluded from the doctors reflections between two consultations. The unconscious and unexpressed emotions and thoughts of doctor and patient are expressed or acted out in the group work.

Luckily the group „thinks aloud". The presenter can follow the process. Emotions are made overt: the patient is uncertain, ambivalent, anxious, stuck…The doctor is stuck, too. He feels helpless, cannot convince the patient and that makes him angry. He is annoyed by the patient and he would prefer not to see him again. On the other hand he wants to help. He might have doubts about the diagnoses and treatment… All this is mentioned in the group.

And sometimes the presenter already has a flash of insight while listening: „Oh, we both feel helpless, are angry, ambivalent, anxious…" When the leaders ask the presenter to move back in and participate he might express his experiences and understanding. Sometimes he adds important details to the story, which he had forgotten to tell – the patient might have done similar in the second consultation. Sometimes he already feels encouraged or relieved,well supported and now begins to understand what is going on between him and the patient.

Questions may stay open

The presenter may feel as helpless as before. The group seems to have worked in vain – an insult, ungratefulness or just the parallel process?

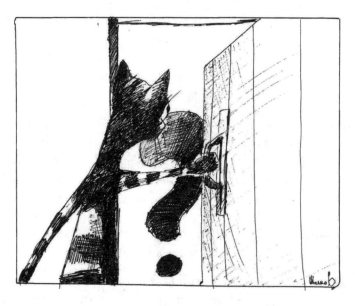

...open question...

The group leader may ask the presenter to push back again, and then reflect in the group, what the feedback meant for their work. How do they all feel when they succeeded? And how does it feel when they seemed to have failed? And of course the group leaders have to find out what the reaction meant to them and their work. Sometimes the group leader is in the doctor's shoes. Just as he felt the frustration with the patient, the group and the leaders are frustrated. They were not able to help, although they tried hard and worked on the case for a long time, more than the doctor and the patient had spent time on it.

It is important to understand the frustration and to put it into the right context.

Example 7. *A GP tells the group, that she is frustrated with a 42 years old patient, who complained of abdominal pain. She has known for 4 years that she has type 1 diabetes mellitus. Her father and brother have a diabetes type 2. When she complains about something at home they reject her by saying that it is not a problem to have diabetes. They can manage, so why can't she. She works in an agency of a health insurance company. Her colleagues do not like it when she does her blood tests at her desk. So she feels rejected, criticized and unwanted there, too.*

She demands a sick leave certificate from her GP, the presenter. The GP asks her for another appointment to do more investigations to make a proper diagnosis related to her symptom — abdominal pain. The patient refuses. The doctor tells her that she will not give her the sick leave certificate when she is not willing to follow her advice. But the GP does not feel comfortable about this intervention, which seems like coercion to her. She asks, „What is going wrong between us?" And that is what the group is working on now.

The group works hard. The members mirror the helplessness, the anger and frustration of the doctor. They are thinking of what they would do, how they could convince the patient or force her ... After a while the presenter comes back and gives her first feedback. The group work did not really help, she did not hear anything new, she still does not feel comfortable when she imagines the patient at the next consultation. The group is frustrated. They thought they had offered a lot but their work seems to have been insufficient.

When the leader points out the parallel process both the group and the presenter smile and are relieved. The presenter feels like the patient, the group did not meet her needs so far.

The group goes on working, stepping into the patients shoes now. What does she want and what would she need? „Nobody understands what a burden my chronic disease is." — „It must have been a shock and very difficult for you four years ago when you got this diagnoses" — somebody said in the GP's shoes.

And suddenly it fell like scales fell from the presenter's eyes. Instead of fighting with the patient and forcing her to undergo more investigations, she could just try to change the perspective. We as doctors see a lot of patients with chronic illnesses. But the individual patient is confronted with her own disease in quite a different way. Her fate is unique, not like that of her father, her brother or other patients. And finally her doctor has understood, appreciated and respected her very special experience.

So a parallel process took place between the doctor patient-relationship and the relationship between the presenter and the Balint group. When the presenter succeeds to identify with the patient and all the accompanying emotions, then from this perspective she will be able to understand the interaction much better.

The group works like a magnifying glass. Every detail is looked at. Every emotion is verbalized. What has happened in 5 minutes during the consultation is now spread out in more than one hour by 8 to 12 experts.

In this process the presenter is in the patient's shoes, the group reflects the doctor's situation and the leaders act like a supervisor, bringing all the aspects to the surface.

7. The Leaders' Training

As we have seen so far, to play the leaders' role requires a lot of experience and knowledge. A group of experienced members may be able to work on their own. One sometimes gets this impression in our training groups. The members have participated in Balint groups and are psychotherapists with professional experience and have learned about group dynamics before. Anyway, it is a challenge for the leader to reflect on his position in the group and his influence on the group work. It is different from leading a group with newcomers or with students. It is different from leading a group of GPs or Psychiatrists or a mixed group. The more experience you have, the more relaxed you can be to do this work, the more interesting it gets. You see all the details and can use the dynamics to help the presenter understand his difficulties.

Requirements to enter the Leaders' Training

Before one enters the Leaders' Seminar you have to have fulfilled certain stages of training. In Germany you have to be a Medical Doctor or a Clinical Psychologist with additional training as Psychotherapist.

In this training you had to have been a member of a self-experience group or you undertook self-experience training in a single setting. You have learned a variety of techniques of Psychotherapy, which you later on can make use of for Balint groups.

And you have to have been a member of a Balint group for 35 sessions. This is one of the important preconditions to enter the training seminar. If it was not part of your training, you have to get your experience in Balint group work in weekend workshops or congresses.

Stages and criteria

International Balint Federation – Basics:

- Leaders should have appropriate basic training, e.g. Family Practitioner, Psychoanalyst, Psychotherapist, Psychologist.

- Leaders should have prior experience of being in a Balint Group.

- Leaders should have worked with an accredited leader for sufficient period of time.

- Leaders should have acquired an understanding of the Doctor-Patient-relationship.

- Leaders should receive adequate supervision.

ALSO Leaders should be able to demonstrate:

- that they create a safe and free environment within the group

- that they focus the work on the Doctor-Patient-relationship rather than seek solutions

- that they create a learning environment rather than resort to didactic teaching.

In Germany we have the following criteria for the leaders' accreditation:

- You have to be a specialist for Psychotherapy, Psychoanalysis, Psychosomatics or Psychiatry for Adults or Children.

- After your specialization you have to have 3 years' experience in your profession plus membership of a Balint group for another 70 sessions. It is desirable to get to know different accredited leaders in this part of the training.

- Then you can start with your training in the Leaders' Seminars. You have to attend 6 seminars with at least 30 sessions, where you get your practical experience and theoretical basics.

- At the same time you are asked to work in a group with an experienced leader as co-leader.

- Psychologists have to have clinical training and additional education as Psychotherapist or Psychoanalyst. Altogether they need 105 sessions of Balint work as a group member.

Classical Balint groups

These are the requirements to lead a classical Balint group.

Classical groups need psychoanalytical thinking. The leader oscillates between emotions and rational thinking, between observation and analysis, between the here and now and the meta position. The parallel process always is in his mind.

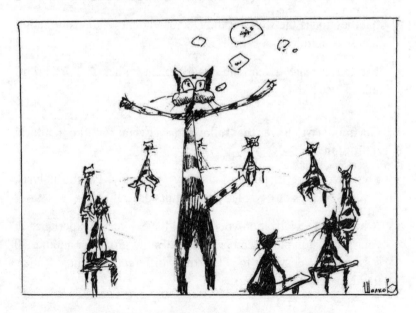

...group process...

The group members work with their empathy and their competence of identifying with other persons. Scenes may appear. The leader verbalizes emotions and points out scenes showing up in the group. His interventions interpret and structure the **group process**.

Balint groups with Sculpture work

Freud put his focus on the intrapsychic conflicts of the patient. Balint considered the interaction mother-child, doctor-patient etc. Today we are also interested in the systemic view. **The sculpture** shows the system of the doctor and the system of the patient, which they live and work in. These systems influence the relationship.

Let us think of a doctor, who is under pressure because he is not allowed to give the best treatment. The patient does not have the money to pay for it, and the health care system cannot afford it.

Imagine a patient who does not dare to take some days off to recover because he might lose his job. All these circumstances affect the doctor-patient relationship. And you can show this to group members, who represent the doctor, the patient, the health care system, the illness, the boss, the family etc.

The leader opens the group work as usual, the presenter tells his story and clarifying questions are asked. It is good to have two leaders when doing sculpture work. The co-leader takes over to build the sculpture together with the presenter.

The presenter chooses the protagonists and positions them in the room. The co-leader will assist him. Attention to body language is most important. Where does the person look? What gesture does he make? Does he turn to or away from the others? Does he touch somebody? When the protagonists are in the assigned position,the presenter gives them one sentence: what is the single person thinking, feeling in this position?

After a moment of silence, during which the protagonists sense and reflect about their positions, the co-leader interviews them. „What are you feeling in this position and this situation with the other people around." „And what would you like to change in the sculpture in order to feel better?"

It is of importance to note which sequence the presenter chooses. All protagonists hear what the others say, how they feel and what changes they wish. This might influence their emotions and wishes. And it is interesting, too, whether the presenter forgets somebody, maybe the patient or himself. All this can be part of the parallel process.

The presenter listens carefully and then chooses one or more people to modify their sculpture. One, two or more people now try to improve their situation. If it is one or two persons, they may change their own position and that of the others. Another possibility is to let them all change and look for a better position in a certain time until the co-leader stops them. Both ways you will get a second sculpture – a significant change and new perspectives.

The presenter and the rest of the group watch the change in all its aspects.

Then the co-leader interviews all the protagonists again. Who is feeling better? Maybe somebody is feeling worse.

It is already the pictures of the two different sculptures that may have an effect on the presenter. Suddenly he understands what makes the relationship so difficult. He is able to change his perspective, finds his way out of the dilemma.

Example 8. *A female Psychotherapist presents a 50 years old female patient with major depression. This patient has a big family and has always worked hard despite the kids having grown up. She takes care of the grand children and supports everybody around. She wants to make it right and please everybody. She is exhausted. The therapist* *feels exhausted as well. She tries to support the patient, giving her positive feedback for all the sacrifices she has made. But nothing changes. The therapist feels like she is supporting the whole system in an unhealthy way and cannot find a way out.*

In the sculpture the patient is sitting in the middle, arms wide open, her husband is besides her but looks in another direction, the others watch her demandingly. The patient expresses that she feels as if she is nailed to the cross. The presenter then asks everybody to look for a better position. The husband leaves for a foreign country. The children are happy to live their own life without anybody controlling them. The grandchildren find grandmas' house empty and look for friends and a playground. And the patient finds a pillar to lean on. She is standing relaxed, wishes arise to enjoy life, erotic phantasies come up. For the presenter scales fall from her eyes. That is the subject they should talk about: pleasure, lust, desire, joy.... detaching from the old patterns and starting a new stage in life.

The sculpture has to be terminated with a ritual. Emotions in the sculpture can be very intense. The roles may weigh heavily on the protagonists, making it especially important to release them from those roles. The presenter turns to every single person, gives him his hand, thanks him for the role and releases him. The co-leader watches this process carefully. When he realizes that a protagonist is still very moved, he cares for him or her. We just experienced this in a group where one of the group members played the role of a child, which had died. She was in tears when the sculpture was terminated. The co-leader very sensibly accompanied her and talked to her until she was able to leave the role behind and come back to her position as a group member. The group then joins in the circle and the leader who started the group work takes over again. A group discussion follows to discuss all aspects.

What does this procedure add to the group work? The use of **body language** deepens the emotional level. The relationship and influences on it are made visible and understandable. The change of scene gives the stimulus for an altered view. It is easier for the presenter to step back and reach the meta position.

The emotions evoked during the process – especially within the protagonists, but also in the spectators – are intense, stay in mind, can be recalled and will influence the doctor-patient communication. Identification with the patient for example is a very special and important **emotional experience** and fosters the ability to change perspectives.

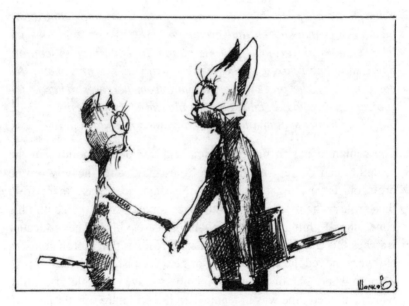

...emotional experience...

The group dynamics is different from the analytical group setting. For a while the discussion group opens up and gives room for the scene of the performance. Intense emotions are evoked and brought back for the discussion and reflection parts. The focus on the presented case is intensified. After the sculpture work the leader comes back to the presenter's matter of concern and the doctor-patient-relationship. „We have heard the presenter's report and we experienced the sculpture work. What are your feelings, your phantasies, your impressions now?" The parallel process is often intensified by sculpture work.

Example 9. *A young intern in training presented a patient she had seen in the outpatient department. He came together with his brother, who pushed him in a wheel chair. The patient had neurological defects. The doctor was not able to say at that point that he understood her questions because his brother always answered. He made strict demands on behalf of his brother that he must have antibiotics because he had cloudy urine. The colleague read in the medical record that the patient should only have antibiotics when he had a fever. In the past he was given too many antibiotics, which did not do any good. She explained this, but the brother insisted. So, she went out of the room to consult one of the senior doctors. He supported her decision to first do more investigations. The brother was furious but had to accept it. This episode was still upsetting the intern.*

In the sculpture we could feel the the narrowness of space and the dominance of the patient's brother. Surprisingly the protagonist, the brother, did not feel superior or demanding in his role, but anxious, uncertain and desperate. In the first sculpture he was the only one standing. In the modified sculpture all three were sitting, and the doctor and patient had eye contact. The situation was far more relaxed.

In the subsequent reflection the group talked about the brother, his attitude, feelings and behavior. The group leader let it go for a while and then she made a remark about having lost the presenter and the patient, who were out of sight. The presenter was thankful for this remark. She listened carefully and had the feeling that she and her concerns were not the focus, but that it was her problem the group was asked to deal with. And she suddenly understood that this was the situation of the patient. In the consultation she was caught in the conflict with the brother, and had lost sight of the patient. And that was what really upset her.

This parallel process, where the presenter experienced the patient's emotions was supported by the sculpture. The brother was dominant in the sculpture and dominated the discussion. The doctor-patient-relationship was repressed, just as it was in the consultation.

The push-back technique added to it. When the presenter was listening to the discussion, not expressing herself, she was close to the patient in his silent role. She now felt for him and focused more on his situation.

For Balint group leaders, who use the above-mentioned additional elements, it is necessary to have experience with these techniques. The training in systemic therapy contains most of these techniques. To prepare for leading this kind of Balint group you have your training in systemic techniques, in classical Balint work and you attend Leaders' Seminars. After leading classical Balint groups you get additional training to lead groups using creative elements. This gives solid grounding. You can then offer different approaches in your groups.

It is important to let the group and the presenter make the choice. With sculpture work the presenter has to cooperate and do more than in a classical Balint group. He is the sculptor. He has to agree to do it. Emotions in these groups are much more intense. When you are in a certain position in the sculpture, you feel the pain, the anxiety, the exhaustion etc. The protagonists express these feelings. The group has to be ready for this experience.

8. What a Balint group Leader should be aware of

In the Balint group leaders' workshops we get an idea of what can go wrong and which behaviour or interventions are not helpful for the presenter. This is a very important ingredient of the training. As Balint said: *„The group leader may make mistakes – in fact he often does – without causing much harm if he can accept criticism in the same or even somewhat sharper terms than he expects his group to accept. .... „ (Balint 1957)* Does this fit together with W. Stuckes observation: *„As a Balint group leader you can do everything, nothing is wrong, you just have to be aware of what you are doing. "*?

We train for both of the above in the Leaders' Seminars. In the feedback part of the session it is important that the leader in training listens to and accepts criticism. That is the essence of the training. Learning by doing means doing it better next time. To get awareness of what was going on you need the feedback from the observer, the presenter and the group members. The leader thus learns to notice what resulted from his interventions during the group process. This is the goal of the training.

In a classical Balint group

Example 10. A young Psychiatrist in training tells the story of a 20 years old patient who is a university student. One day people found the patient almost naked close to a river; he claimed that his father had punished him and he had run away. He was brought to the psychiatric clinic by the police. The experienced colleagues diagnosed a psychoses and prescribed medication. The presenter was uncertain. He tended to believe the patient. He wanted to know more about the father-son-relationship, but he did not get an opportunity to find out. With these uncertainties he presented the case.

The group leader was an experienced psychiatrist. His introductory intervention to open the group work was: „We have a young presenter and a young patient where the presenter suspects a father-son-conflict. What are your thoughts about that?" You could feel his intention to lead the group to convince the presenter that the experienced psychiatrists were right.

The group leader tended to move the group members in a certain direction. In this way he was narrowing the phantasies, free associations and emotions. In the following discussion the leader stressed statements, which supported the diagnosis „Psychosis" and ignored others about the father-son-relationship.

Luckily there was a co-leader, who took care of the presenter, brought him back in early and asked him about his feelings. The presenter said: „Most of you do not believe me. But I am sure there is a conflict. Maybe both are true. He has a psychosis and there is a bad father-son-relationship, which is important to him."

In the feedback the group and the observers pointed out the parallel process. The presenter had felt the rejection just like the patient. He was able to verbalize his disappointment. Fortunately there was a co-leader who took him seriously. The leader had a hypothesis right away and tried to bring the group in his direction. He was not open to other possibilities. He became aware, during the feedback dicsussion, of his attitude and his narrowing of the process with his first intervention.

The feedback, which the leader gets during his training, is in accord with what the doctor gets as a presenter in the Balint group: how do my emotions and my attitude influence the relationship/group process. I learn a lot about myself, my emotions, my prejudices, my projections, my transference and countertransference.

In this case it helped to identify the parallel process during the feedback. In a regular Balint group this would probably not have been the case. The presenter might have gone home with the feeling:

„Maybe I was wrong. But they did not understand what bothered me. The Balint group did not really help me." The experience in the group might have been the same experience as in the clinic. He would not have come to a broader view. In the leaders' training group he now understood that it was ok to give antipsychotic medication. As well he wanted to talk to the patient again, take him seriously and find out about his relationship with his father.

Another important issue is **„the question to the group"**. Leaders tend to ask the presenter at the end of his report: „Would you please formulate a question to the group." This could be a temptation misleading the group. The question to the group often is: „What would you do in this situation" or „What shall I do with the patient?" The temptation is the word „do".

In Balint work our focus is on the relationship, transference and countertransference, with all the associated emotions, with prejudice, with blind spots, with ignorance… The „to do" questions keep the group away from the essence. Good advice will follow, practical hints, solutions for the future handling of the case.

A helpful invitation to the presenter maybe: "Would you please give a short summary of your problem with the patient." – „Well, when I see his name shining up in my computer I already feel an unwillingness to care for him, and I don't know why."

As the focus is the relationship, you usually do not need a question or summary at all. „What is going on between the two persons?" is always the assignment in the room.

In a Balint group with Sculpturing

Example 11. *Frauke, one of the young GPs, presented a case:*

An elderly couple, in their mid-sixties, dropped into her consulting room. The woman complained of swollen feet; her shoes would not fit any more. Frauke was shocked when she examined her. Water was running out of ulcers on her legs. Her abdomen was filled with ascites and her liver was firm. She had a blood test the next day. As she expected she found signs of liver cirrhosis. She could smell the alcohol when the couple first stepped into her room. Frauke tried to convince them that the woman had to go to hospital for further investigations and treatment. They refused. The mother of the patient had her 85th birthday the following Sunday, and the patient had promised to bake her a cake. She insisted, that she could not now tell her mother that she could not bake her a cake. Frauke noticed that both did not understand how serious the situation was. They repeated that they just wanted the shoes to fit again. She had the impression that the husband was the one who blocked the patient's acceptance. So, she decided to see the patient alone next time and to convince her. She likes the patient and pities her. She does not like the husband very much. She wants to find out how best to help the patient.

The leader offers her the opportunity to build a sculpture and she agrees:

Susanne – a doctor working in a Psychosomatic clinic – is the patient.

Johannes — working in a psychiatric clinic – is the husband.

Christiane – also working in a Psychosomatic clinic – is the doctor.

Heike – a specialist in orthopedics – is the 85-year-old mother of the patient.

Frauke, the presenter, brings the actors into positions she thinks would fit. Then she steps behind everybody and gives him or her one sentence: that which she she feels or thinks is appropriate for them and their positions.

The patient: "I don't understand what is wrong with me; I just want to function like ever."

The husband: "I hope you can make her fit again."

The mother: "My birthday is coming up and my daughter will of course take care of all I need."

The doctor: "I want to help her."

Of course, we are aware that all those thoughts represent the doctor's inner picture of the situation. And that is our chance to change the focus, create alternatives and enlighten her blind spots. Frauke, the presenter, now looks at the scene from a distance. The first scales fall from her eyes. She suddenly understands the patient's situation as she observes it and her own emotional reaction.

The sculpture shows, that mother, husband and doctor were dragging the patient to different sides.

The next step is to ask the actors how they feel in their position, and how they would like to change the scene to feel better. It is the group leader's task to interview the protagonists. It is very important to ask an open question without provoking a particular answer.

The leader asks: „How do you feel in this position?" and not for examplel:„Isn't that a difficult position you are in? Should you not care better for yourself, for your health?" — which would be a closed question; the patient has only the choice to say „Yes" or „No".

The patient answers the open question that she feels under pressure and does not know whom to trust and whom to follow. She does not take her illness seriously. Her big belly and swollen feet bother her; she just wants to get rid of these symptoms to function better again. Her problem is that she is not able to serve both: her husband and her mother. She wishes to sit with the doctor and her husband and discuss what to do next.

A possible closed question to the husband could be: „Don't you see, how ill your wife is?" The open question: „How do you feel?" gives much more information.

The husband feels bothered and angry that his everyday life is disturbed, that he does not have his wife just for himself and that she has problems. He wants to take her with him and leave doctor and mother behind. Alcohol had always been a good solution for all problems; he trusts this experience more than the doctor.

A closed question for the mother could be: „Are you aware of the problems your daughter has?" To the open question: „How do you feel?" she answers, that she is irritated that her daughter turned away from her and that a doctor is in the room. She wants her to look in her direction and just take notice of her and nobody else.

The doctor expresses her discomfort; she wants to be alone with the patient, excluding the mother and husband.

Frauke, the presenter, listens carefully.

Then the leader asks her to make a decision as to whom she wants to give the opportunity to change the scene. Frauke chooses the patient.

In the second sculpture — now created by the patient — the patient, her husband and the doctor sit together in a triangle. And these are the answers the leader gets in his interviews to the open questions: The patient cannot see her mother; she feels relief. The new situation is also better for the doctor. The husband is not content but he can accept the change. The mother is angry, disappointed and anxious.

Afterwards the group went on with the group discussion as usual. The sculpturing takes about 10 to 15 minutes. We always take 90 minutes to work on one case. If you have two leaders it could be wise to ask the other leader to now lead the discussion. He was able to watch the sculpturing from a distance and was not involved in the scene.

He may start with a question to the presenter: „Having experienced the sculpture, did your question to the group change?"

Or he may start with an intervention addressing the group: „You remember the story and you have attended the sculpting process. What are your feelings, thoughts and phantasies about this doctor-patient-relationship?"

The group discussion afterwards is vivid, with less rationalization or good advice. Emotions are felt and not only thought about. Of course, it is the doctor-patient-relationship on which we focus and the leader reminds the group of this once in a while.

Frauke gets a different point of view about her relationship. She understands that she does not have to be a rival to the mother or husband to save the patient. She is able to watch the scene from a distance and feel her unrealistic demands. She is now able to accept the situation, taking it as it is and try to make the best out of it. She feels sadness and a small glimpse of hope. She is impressed; even her feelings towards the husband has changed during the process. His presence does not bother her any more. She expresses her curiosity to see the patient again.

The sculpture has side effects, too.

Johannes, the young psychiatrist, is surprised because he experienced that, being in the shoes of the patient's husband, he did not recognize the destroying power of the alcohol of himself and his partner. Nobody would have been able to tell him. In real life he, as a Psychiatrist, has tried to convince his patients of the negative effect of alcohol and drugs on body and mind and is disappointed when he was not successful, as when the addicts did not follow his arguments. In the sculpture he feels the denial.

Susanne, as the patient, is aware of her defences not to accept being very ill. She has to be present and fit for her mother and her husband, who both denied her illness as well. For her this is a new experience.

Christiane, as the doctor, feels the tension, horror and anger in this situation. At the same time, she is professional and wants to help, although she feels the limits to her success. Her first impulse is to say: leave the alcohol, change your life completely, and get out of your dependency. Then she understands that this is not possible for this patient, that this family lives in a quite different world with different goals and intentions than she does.

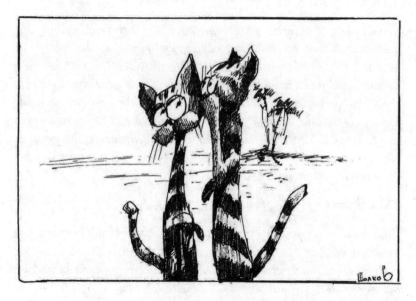

...*message of the doctor to the patient...*

Her first impulse is to give **a message to the patient** in her (what Balint called) „**apostolic function**", „which means in the first place that every doctor has a vague, but almost unshakably firm idea of how a patient ought to behave when ill". (Balint 1957).

The actors in the sculpture develop intense emotions. It is a strengthening of empathy and self-experience for each of them, which does not have to be verbalized in details; it will stay with them.

In the discussion afterwards we could use their emotional experiences to better understand the situation. And, of course, the onlookers add their observations and emotions to the discussion.

It is the task of the leaders to make use of the expressed emotions, bringing the protagonists back to the meta position and focussing on the doctor-patient relationship with all its external influences.

We are aware that what we set in scene is the perception of the presenter. It is subjective and shows the emotions of the presenter evoked by the patient and the system in which they live. Sculpturing gives a chance to play with reality, to open up to different views and new thoughts, to have a healthy distance and (not seldomly) get back to smiles, laughter and good humor – in spite of all the difficulties in the case, the working facilities and, last but not least, in the health care system.

The group meets again a few weeks later and the leader asks for feedback. Frauke reports that she was quite surprised when the patient came to her next appointment without her husband. She was well dressed, clean and without the smell of alcohol. It seemed like a miracle "as if the patient had been present in the group discussion..." Frauke herself was curious and happy to see the patient. She was able to support the patient with her own possibilities, just like the group had supported her and not force the patient with „good advice" or moral appeal.

9. Leading different groups

One of our accredited leaders once told me: „It is much more difficult than I thought to work with groups outside the training. It is quite different from what I experienced in the Leaders' Seminars" That is true. In the Leaders' Seminars you work with advanced experienced colleagues, who had training in psychological thinking. In „real life" you work with groups of layman in this sense. And this was Balint's goal: „the psychologizing of doctoring" as he called it.

As group leaders we work with helping professions, who mostly are not used to this kind of analytical reflection and analyzing relationships in this way.

Homogeneous or heterogeneous groups

Michael Balint started in London with a group of GPs. He was asked to help them understand patients with psychosomatic reactions after the Second World War. Balint and his first wife Alice had previously experimented with groups in Budapest. Now he wanted to teach psychosomatics and at the same time study the pharmacology of the drug „doctor". He called his group „Training cum Research Group in Relationship" – to train the doctors in psychosomatic knowledge, diagnosis and treatment and to get to know more about the effects of the doctor on his patient and the effect of the doctor-patient-relationship on diagnosis and treatment. „The doctor as a drug".

To work with only GPs in the group has advantages and disadvantages. The group members with the same profession have a lot of experience in common. You need not explain difficulties with home visits or with non-compliant patients, who come back again and again with new complaints. They all know about this. On the other hand, your group members' thoughts may go in the same direction. Somebody from a different profession may look at it from another angle and throw light on blind spots. Homogeneous groups may have the same defences.

Balint's idea was to discuss the psychological aspects of the GP's everyday practice. He, as a psychiatrist, knew more about the background of psychosomatic diseases and the interface between body and soul. But he did not want to **teach** the group, he wanted the GPs to find out about the underlying emotions. Just as the psychotherapist does not teach his client and helps him understand his conflicts.

In a homogenous group the members have comparable experiences and difficulties with patients and with the setting. Their professional identity, self-image and self-understanding are similar. That may help them concentrate on the case presentation and on the doctor's needs. But it could also evoke a common defence. As the experiences with the work situation and the health care system are about the same, individual problems with certain patients and the patient's perspective could easily be projected on these circumstances. Thus the self experience part could be dropped and new perspectives narrowed. The development of the individual participant, which has been evaluated in research projects, will probably not occur, unless the group leader is a specialist with a psychotherapeutic background – just like Balint was. He then indicates and leads the participants to an understanding of the individual conflict, e.g. in the case when the doctor wanted the patient to have more investigations. A homogenous group might have agreed with forcing her to do so and thought of ways to succeed in this. In the above example group, work changed and developed after the group leader brought the presenter back and she was able to express her frustration. After that the parallel process enabled group members to step into the patient's shoes. „Nobody understands what a burden my chronic disease is". This is much easier for a group member who is not confronted with similar problems in his daily professional life. In a homogenous group the group leader himself often has to shift the focus to the patient's perspective.

In a group with different specialists and professions this possibility is minimized. Critical reflections are possible; the view of an outsider helps. The patient's perspective becomes easier. The disadvantage of a heterogenous group might be that more misunderstandings occur, which need to be cleared up. But sometimes these questions for better understanding lead to a flash, which enlightens the presenter to the problem. They are interesting for other kinds of specialists.

For the Balint group leader it is most important that he has enough **field competence** to follow the presenter's and the group members' rational and emotional statements.

With physicians, psychologists, psychiatrists

A mixed group brings a lot of interesting perspectives and views from different angles. There is various identification with the different people in the presenter's story. It seems to be easier to step into the shoes of the patient and his family when you are not in the

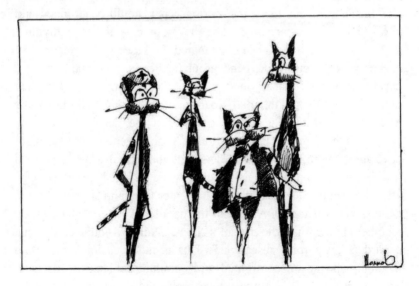

...mixed groups...

same profession. A psychiatrist has a different view on the patient than the GP or the gynaecologist or a student. You often experience anger arising when you do not quite understand what is going on in the other person, for example the patient. When you find a reasonable explanation the anger vanishes. Empathy is an important prerequisite for this kind of understanding. You train your empathy even more in a group with different people, different patients and different stories.

The leader of a mixed group learns a lot from other professions. He trains his openness, tolerance, respect and eagerness. As a leader you are always aware that you work with different experts in the group. You are the expert for group dynamics and analytical thinking. The group members are experts in their fields.

With students

Balint, in the first place, did not want to work with students in his groups. He thought they were not mature enough to resonate with the doctor-patient-relationship. It was Boris Luban-Plozza who convinced him that students, with their views not yet spoiled by routine and frustration, have an inspiring influence on the group's work. They are able to have free associations, to think fresh and to let phantasies blossom. Their often idealistic views of their desired professions bring valuable perspectives to the realistic, sometimes pessimistic attitudes of experienced professionals. Mixed groups bring doctors and students together and both can learn a lot from each other.

Groups with only students also work perfectly. They mostly bring relief to the students who meet patients for the first time. They learn that they are not alone with their uncertainty, their struggles and criticism. Students are not yet doctors and they are not patients. They are in between. When they describe their problems with patients it is often their identification with, for example a young dying patient or trauma patient. That is what they can imagine. The doctor's role is still strange and uneasy for them, not yet familiar and fully accepted. Criticism of the medical system, the practice of medicine and about medicare is worth listening to. Ideas for improving the training of medical students may come up.

Example 12. A student in his 3rd year in Medical School has a placement in a surgical department. He is instructed to take the history from a patient and do a physical examination before surgery. Together with a colleague he waits outside the hospital room. One of the surgeons passes by and asks them: „What are you looking for? – oh, sorry, I forgot, you are here to examine one of the patients for your course. I have no time right now, please, wait here." One hour later: "Oh, you are still here. Didn't anybody look after you and take you to the patient? I will send somebody to do that." another 1 1/2 hour later: „Come on, I will quickly help you to see the patient. I know the time of your seminar is over." They enter a room. A 70 year old patient, pale and anxious is lying in his bed. The doctor approaches him quickly, moves his blanket, points to his abdomen and invites the students to inspect and examine it. The students hesitate, they feel ashamed. How can they step over the patient's border just like that. „I am Frank. Sorry, is it ok with you that I just have a look? And may I touch your body?" The patient keeps quiet but nods. Frank can feel a big tumor in the epigastric. „Now what is it?" the surgeon asks impatiently. „I feel a tumor in the epigastric:"- „Yes, right, this patient has pancreatic cancer. We will take care of it tomorrow. Not a big chance for cure, but we can try. You can come to watch the operation? I have to go now. If you have some extra time, talk to the patient, take his story. I will give you my signature anyway. See you tomorrow." The two students stay behind and are shocked. When they look at the patient, they see tears in his eyes. What to do? „Is it ok with you if we ask some questions or would you rather be alone?" Frank asks. „Thank you for asking, but I would rather be alone." They both leave him with very bad feelings.

The group is agitated, touched and angry. Most of them are immediately in the patient's shoes, others express their empathy with Frank. What a terrible situation. Has anybody talked to the patient before? Or was he just treated like this all the time? How brutal can medical care be? And why are medical students treated like that? They feel burdensome, unnecessary, redundant. But they are the future doctors. Why are the present doctors not interested in doing their very best to pass on their knowledge? They understand that a surgeon has a hard and tiring job. But is that an excuse or an explanation to treat patients and students like that? Frank feels better with being accepted and understood. All students in the group are sure that they will handle similar situations differently during their careers. There is hope that they will remember this Balint group.

One of the important points is definitely to learn more about the effect of talking to patients and listening to their stories.

For the Balint group leader it is important to notice what kind of difficulties students talk about in Balint groups.

We found four recurring themes in Balint work with medical students in the last year before graduation from University:

a. Problems the students are having in their own socialization during medical training.

b. The role of the student during his practical year at the university hospital.

c. Struggles with the ideal image of being a doctor and the reality.

d. The wish and need for self-exploration through the Balint group experience.

Leading student groups has some special features. The doctor or psychologist leading is often either perceived as representative of the clinic and the medical establishment or simply as an opponent of the rational side of somatic medicine. Sometimes he is idealized as the doctor who is aware of his own emotional reactions and possibilities; at the same time, he takes good care of the patient's physical and his emotional concerns with a holistic view.

In the Balint group students deal with their struggle with everyday realities in clinical work, which they experience as insufficient and annoying. After a while they become more tolerant, realistic and get a more nuanced picture of an idealistic and a feasible approach to the patient, with the focus on both sides: the rational and the emotional, the somatic and the psychological. The leader is reminded of his own struggles in his student life. It maybe an advantage to keep the balance between teaching and letting go of the experience.

The International Balint Federation (IBF) together with the Foundation Psychosomatics and Social Medicine award a prize every second year for medical students with their essays describing a student-patient-relationship – their reflections about it and about the medical training and the healthcare system in their part of the world. Some of these student essays from the last almost 40 years have been published. They give an interesting insight into the students' experiences during their medical training in different countries over the years.

With members of other helping professions

We refer to groups in which helpers from different occupations are gathered, such as physicians, psychologists, nurses, social workers, ergo-therapists, medical assistants, physiotherapist, music therapists, hospital chaplains and teachers. The pre-condition and understanding in these groups is that every participant is willing to be truly involved in the clarifying process and to contribute stories of their own difficult relationships. Another very important condition is confidentiality: everything that is said in the group stays in the group and is not discussed elsewhere.

The different perspectives introduced by group members from their real experiences in their field can make a substantial contribution to clarification and enlightenment. As in the Balint groups with different specialists the leader needs tolerance, respect and understanding of their various fields. It is a challenge and an enrichment for his own profession.

Different cultural background and nationalities

Today it is an everyday experience to have Balint groups with members with different cultural backgrounds. At the same time the presented patients are from different nationalities as well. As a Balint group leader you are lucky to have group members who are able to explain behaviours, beliefs and typical anxieties which are due to the various backgrounds. As Balint put it: „the group leader should not be the smartest member of the group" He is the one who collects and values the statements. As a leader you learn a lot from group members. Prejudices are welcome to make them open. This way you learn about your own errors in perception. „All teachers are narrow minded", „All people from the countryside are naive" .... you will find a lot of examples in the group. It is wise to think about your own prejudices as a leader and maybe correct them.

Example 13. *The psychiatrists in training in a psychiatric clinic meet in a Balint group. It is an obligatory part of their development as specialists. In this group there are colleagues from Russia, Ukraine, Turkey, Iran, Poland and Germany. One Turkish trainee presents a case: the patient is a 43 years old male. He grew up in a Turkish village, moved to Germany when he was 18 years old and has lived in an arranged marriage since then. He works as a craftsman in a small company. He has two daughters, 16 and 18 years old. He describes himself as becoming very aggressive since being married.*

He often quarrelled with his wife, beat her, was not much at home, spent a lot of money gambling and did not care for his children. When his father died in 2009 he suddenly became afraid of going to hell. He became religious and made a pilgrimage to Mecca. When he came back he was a nice father and a good husband. He went to the Mosque and prayed regularly. His life changed completely. When he came to the Psychiatric clinic 7 years later he was depressed. He said that he was suffering from aggressive outbursts, had inner unrest, sleep disorder and anxiety for the previous two years. When his mother died in 2013 he had a nervous breakdown. Since then he had visions of different characters – he calls them Dschinn – who determine his life events. They are there – he can see them – and they tell him what to do. He does not dare to oppose them. Some of those Dschinns are nice, others torture him.

The presenter is of Turkish origin, and he grew up with Dschinns as well. He explains to the group that in the Muslim faith these are supernatural creatures who live with us, but are usually invisible to us and only in special situations do they become visible. When he was a kid, the grown ups warned him: „Watch out, the Dschinns see and know everything you do.“ Now the presenter does not know what to think. Was this patient paranoid? Or was this magic thinking? He tried to convince the patient that the Dschinns lived just in his fantasy, although he emotionally was not quite sure; of course he was rational. But the patient was stubborn. Psychotrophic medication did not help. The presenter feels helpless and uncertain.

In the group discussion the group members from different cultural background pretty soon look at the patient as a little boy. They themselves had fantasized figures like that: a bad guy under the bed, an angel above. The parents had supported the good characters, the angels. They look after you, they protect you, they are always with you. Whereas the bad characters are just in your fantasy. But the bad figures were necessary, too. Sometimes parents used these figures: the bad man in the woods who would come and get the naughty children, or father Christmas who gives presents to the good ones and beats the bad ones. Similar stories were told in all cultures.

The bad figures were helpful in a way; hey took over the aggressive emotions and wishes. It was not the little boy who pinched his brother, broke an ear from his beloved teddybear or stole his sisters chocolate bar – it was the nasty figures. It takes a while to integrate our nasty parts. This patient maybe had dis-integrated them. He had repressed or split off all the emotions which did not fit with his new religious life. And he had used the Dschinns to shift the unwanted emotions to them. The presenter remained somewhat sceptical, but took new ideas home. Had the doctor-patient-relationship been like a father with his 5 years old boy? Was that the transference and countertransference?

Six weeks later the presenter gave feedback: He had changed the setting with the patient; they had taken walks where they discussed politics and other apects of reality. They had been more at eye level this way. The patient then was open to arguments and showed an understanding of his situation. He did not talk much about the Dschinns and when he did mentioned them he was not anxious any more. And when they laughed at him he thought: „Wait and see. I will succeed.“ The psychiatrist had the impression that the patient was more mature and improved with creating a distance to his childlike and magical thinking. The psychiatrist now felt more like a partner than a father as he had done before.

Between structuring and letting go, different styles for different groups

As I have worked with many different groups: students, GPs, psychiatrists, gynaecologists, teachers, young doctors, mixed groups, groups in the Psychosomatic Basic Training, groups at weekend workshops, advanced groups, inexperienced groups, groups in China, in Russia, in Romania…., in International Conferences, in IBF

Congresses….. I would not say I am always the same leader. I act according to my impressions as to what would bring the group forward. The main question for me is: „How much structuring does this group need?"

Free associations and fantasies need room. Experienced groups should have a lot of room, they do not need many oral interventions; body language of the leader often does it. They need the safe atmosphere, attentive support and a clear time limit. Inexperienced groups need much more. An intervention may sometimes be an interpretation, or a question, or a provocation to open up new aspects. There is no need to make corrections or evaluate statements. Questions to participants may enlighten the scene. „Why do you think …" or „What is behind your remark?" – „What are you feeling?" Not seldomly the answer is „I think …" And the leader asks again: „What are you feeling?" Medical people are so used to being rational, which is from their training. This is, of course, very meaningful and useful for everyday life. It is not easy to switch from this routine to another perspective.

Students often tend to open up right away and talk about their emotions, their private life and their background. Here the leader is bound to limit the openness in order protect the individual. Sometimes this is the case in long-standing Balint groups as well. It tends to become more and more a self-experience group. Over the years the group members get to know each other well, may have private contacts and have heard many similar stories from the same person about their doctor-patient-relationships. Then it may already be obvious what the difficulties of this colleague are the kinds of patients with whom he has problems. That could make it difficult to stay open to new ideas. The group may develop common defences and common blind spots. Hopefully the leader does not go with them and continues to look from the meta position.

10. Supervision for Balint group Leaders

As a Balint group leader it is important to get feedback on your group work, which is always work in progress, life-long learning. Not only in the beginning of our careers most of us have the desire to exchange thoughts with other leaders, to reflect on the process, to talk about difficulties with individual members, with a group situation, with difficult stories or conflict between the two leaders. Maybe one has a problem with and wants to know how to establish a new group. This exchange with other group leaders is a benefit.

Where can Balint group leaders find help with their problems? Of course it should be possible to phone another leader or, in the first place, discuss the problem with the co-leader.

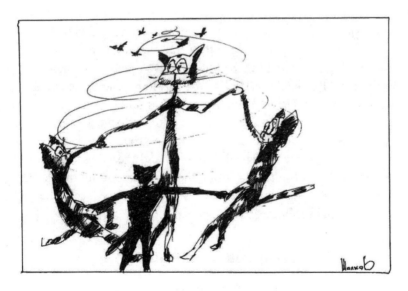

...supervision for leaders...

Supervision of a group at work

To have an observer sitting outside the group while the group is working is one of the possibilities for supervision. We use this method in the leaders' training and in demonstration fishbowls at weekend workshops, where we discuss the process, the group dynamics and the leaders' attitude and interventions openly after the group work. Of course you can always ask another experienced group leader to support you in this way. In many countries this is part of the leaders' training. Experienced leaders observe a Balint group at work with usual group members, who are not trainees themselves.

We often hear the argument that it is so different and more difficult to lead a group outside the training. In the leaders' workshops you have group members who are very experienced themselves. In Germany they attended about 100 group sessions as members, had a training as psychotherapists and are working with patients in their professions. They all had self-experience training and knowledge of group dynamics. Later on when they lead Balint groups with somatic doctors from different specialities it is a quite challenging new experience. Remember, Balint's goal was to psychologize doctoring. He worked with GPs to research and train the „doctor as a drug", the influence of the personality of the doctor on the patient, on diagnoses and treatment in somatic medicine. Those group members have not had training in psychological thinking. And the cases they present are mostly a lot different from those presented in the leaders' workshops. There is a need to get a supervisor's feedback when you start working with these groups „in real life".

A Supervision group with a facilitator

From time to time it is helpful to meet in a supervision group for Balint group leaders. Usually a facilitator organizes and moderates these groups. You can either work as a self-help group or as a Balint group, where a group or a group member is presented as a „patient".

You then have a story, the questioning round and the discussion with free associations, phantasies and identifications. As in the doctor-patient relationship you may find blind spots in the group leader-presenter, or group leader - group member relationship.

Example 14. *Six experienced Balint group leaders sit together with a facilitator for supervision. They decide to handle the setting like a Balint group. One of them presents a case/group. The others first listen carefully, then may ask clarifying questions. Then the presenter is in the pushback position and comes back after a while.*

One of the group members presents his group in a psychiatric clinic. It consists of 12 members, but mostly 6 to 8 and seldomly 10 are present. They are all psychiatrists in training. The group work takes place at the end of a day, half in working time, half in their free time. Often the participants are tired. But they like doing Balint work with fantasies, thoughts, humor and laughter. The only thing that irritates the group leader is when the members do not arrive on time. He understands that it is sometimes hard to keep on time. But he is unhappy with this situation. What goes wrong between him and the group? This sounds quite familiar to most of the participants of the supervision group. Medical doctors are always busy. They come rushing into the group and even fall asleep during group work. They have night calls and see many patients each day. On top of that they are in training and have extra courses and seminars. The facilitator remarks that they are all very understanding and nice. Was there only empathy with the young colleagues? Somebody said: „No, it makes me angry, too. I wish my Balint group would be so worthwhile that they want to enjoy it from the first to the last moment." – and somebody else adds: „I have to organize my day as well and I am always on time. Why can't they?" The discussion goes on in this direction. Memories of their own training arise when they had strict rules to follow. Of course they sometimes hated it and wished to escape.

The presenter suddenly feels: „Oh, I want the group to love me! I am generous and want to give them joy after their hard work, like a good father. But I do not give them enough structure, which they would need badly for their work-life-balance. I should be a better example and demand something, instead of hiding my anger from them." The participants then discussed how they would tell the group. The anger had vanished now as they had detected it. Maybe you could ask for the group members' solidarity. Some were always on time, the Leader was always on time, how could they manage? What would be the benefit for all of them to start all together?

Supervision groups usually meet at weekend workshops. They offer stimulation for new ideas and for a change. Usually there is no feedback. Anyway, it is a relief to talk about the difficulties and get different perspectives and support in the group. And just as in a usual Balint group the effect multiplies; everybody has similar experiences.

As well, the participants may talk about general questions like: how do you form a new group? Would you serve tea or coffee? What influence might this have on the group work? What would you refuse to be discussed in a Balint group? And how would you do it? If a group member leaves a session what do you do? Would you talk with a member after the session when you feel there is a problem? How do you manage a situation which weighs on you as a leader?

A lot more questions may come up. It is good to have an exchange about them.

An inter-vision group

Another possibility is what we call „inter-vision groups". Some leaders gather without a facilitator and talk about their groups.

Both ways help to establish high quality leadership of Balint groups.

To summarize the conditions for supervision:

Level 1: Participation in a Balint group

Level 2: Participation in a Leaders' Seminar

Level 3: Leading a Balint group under supervision

Level 4: Participation in a supervision group for Balint group leaders

Objective Level 3: an experienced Balint group leader observes a group session of a „normal Balint group" and gives feedback on the group process, the parallel process, the influence of the leaders' attitudes and interventions.

Objective Level 4: Exchange of experiences of difficult situations in Balint groups at home with other Balint group leaders with mutual assistance. This can be done without a facilitator as an intervision group or with a facilitator as a supervision group.

Contents Level 4: A continuum of practical and organizational questions up to the psychodynamics in the group and the processing of the counter transference of the leader.

When does a leader introduce his group?

- Difficulty understanding what is happening in the group.

- Group development is experienced as a burden and unsatisfactory.

- Group leader doubts his competence.

- Disturbances which do not represent the case-dynamics – the parallel process.

Causes of counter transference in the leader:

1. Life experiences, situations that are difficult to cope with and which are triggered in the group.

Goal: To regain safety by self-reflection and at the same time concentrating on the reflections in the group. Luckily your co-leader can help in this process.

2. The bias of the leader. The group does not develop because of the leader's resistance, e.g. against fears, aggression and feelings of insufficiency.

Goal: To bring negative defended emotions into awareness and to name them. Again the co-leader can be helpful.

Practical and organizational questions:

- Forming a new group.

- How to deal with difficult participants?

- Cooperation of co-leaders.

- Group size and session frequency.

- Mix of group participants.

- How to start a group session.

- Observing the group participants.

- Protection of the presenter and the other group members.

- Boundaries of self-experience.

- How much structure does a Balint group session need?

- How to select a case (several offers by different group members).

- How, when and why to refuse a case (offer of a professional relationship e.g. in teams).

11. The Leaders' Tasks

In general

- to create a safe atmosphere;

- to focus on the doctor-patient-relationship / the professional relationship;

- to encourage ideas, phantasies, associations, the expression of emotions and body sensations, dialogues, scenes, role-play;

- to offer an interpretation of scenic encounters, of the group process and the parallel process;

- to differentiate between the case dynamics and the group dynamics, especially disturbances from other sources, which have priority;

- to be aware of one's own emotions, transference and countertransference;

- to promote new perspectives;

- to stimulate empathy and interest;

- to serve as a role model in tolerance, keeping boundaries, listening, finding a balance between structuring and letting go, free floating attention, thoughtfulness.

The Leaders' Role in a Sculpture Group

- the leader opens the group work as usual;

- after clarifying questions the co-leader asks the presenter to choose his protagonists;

- the co-leader assists building the sculpture;

- the co-leader interviews the persons in the sculpture;
- the co-leader asks the presenter to choose somebody to change the sculpture;
- the co-leader interviews the protagonists again;
- the co-leader takes care of the ritual which terminates the sculpture work;
- the co-leader accompanies the protagonists leaving their roles back to their work as group members;
- the leader facilitates the subsequent discussion.

The Leaders follow the Aim of Sculpturing:

- to get to the emotional level by using body language;
- to make the doctor-patient relationship and their system – they live and work in – visible and noticeable;
- to work for the presenter widening his perspective;
- to take care of the protagonists;
- to give the stimulus for an altered view;
- to relieve the presenter;
- to regain interest in the patient;
- to promote the pleasure of doctoring.

The Leaders are aware of the Side-Effects:

- nearly every group member has experienced similar difficult patients and situations;
- emotions evoked during the process stay and can be recalled;

- identification with persons in the sculpture has a self-experience aspect, which stays silent and is not discussed;

- emotions may be intense and need sensible handling;

- the image of the sculpture stays in mind and influences the doctor-patient communication;

- the protagonists may win a self-experience aspect, which they must not share with the group.

12. Conclusion

It sounds quite exhausting to be in the position of the Balint group leader. The good news is the leader has time for reflection while the group is working.

We usually take 90 minutes for the group process dealing with one relationship. That gives the possibility of listening carefully in a relaxed way to the presenter and to the group and to oscillate from the emotional level to the meta position and back.

When the group starts working the leader can focus on her own emotions and discover her own hypotheses concerning the relationship. At the same time, she listens to the opinions and watches the presenter's reactions.

As in psychotherapy our transference, countertransference, empathy and emotional reactions are the instruments with which we work as a Balint group leader. That is why self-experience training is desirable before starting the leaders' training. Knowledge about group dynamics is necessary as we are working with a group.

When you introduce additional elements into your Balint group work you have to complete extra training. This is necessary for all the mentioned techniques: sculpture, psychodrama, imagination and role play. These are techniques taken from psychotherapeutic work. They need to be adapted for use in Balint group work. Special workshops offer these techniques. Life long learning is a valuable principle. For Balint group leaders this means to use supervision or inter-vision in order to exchange and discuss experiences, difficulties and new ideas.

The essence of Balint work, to analyze professional relationships with the goal of professional development and development of instruments to improve interactions, is today not only used for the medical professions, but also for other helping professions such as teachers, lawyers etc.

A Balint group leader needs to gain experience and competence in these different applications of Balint group work.

13. Literature

Balint M (1972) The Doctor, His Patient and the Illness, International Universities Press, Inc., New York.

Flatten G, Möller H, Tschuschke V (2015) Designing the doctor-patient relationship – How beneficial are Balint groups and for whom? Proceedings of the 1st International Balint Conference, Yerevan.

Otten H (2012) Professionelle Beziehungen. Springer, Berlin Heidelberg.

Otten H, Petzold ER (2015) The Student, the Patient and the Illness 2015, Berlin.

Otten,H. Bergmann, G., Nease, D. The Student, the Patient and the Illness 2017, Psychosozial-Verlag, Gießen.

Petzold ER, Otten H (2010) The Student, the Patient and the Illness, Xlibri.

14. Appendix

International Balint Federation – Guidelines for Accreditation of Balint Leaders

These guidelines are intended as parameters for national societies to consider when drawing up their criteria for accreditation. National societies will want to define periods of sufficient lengths of time, for instance being in a Balint Group. Societies need to be aware that it is equally important for psychiatrists and psychotherapists to acquire experience of lleading Balint groups before becoming accredited, as it is for GPs. Although the pathway for psychiatrists and psychotherapists will be different to the pathway for GPs.

1. Leaders should have appropriate basic professional training.

2. Leaders must have prior experience of being in a Balint Group for a sufficient* length of time.

3. Leaders should have co-led with an accredited leader as part of their training. That accredited leader is invited to provide a report/reference to the accrediting society.

4. Leaders should have a supervisor who has sufficient** knowledge of their work to be able to provide a report/reference to the accrediting society.

5. Leaders should be evaluated prior to accreditation according to the following criteria:

   - that they encourage the development of a safe and free environment within the group and are aware of the importance of protecting the boundaries of the group;

   - that they focus the work on an exploration of the doctor-patient relationship rather than seeking solutions or teaching;

- that they are open to learning about their personal style in leading a group and aware that their attitudes and responses will influence the dynamics of the group;

- that they have an awareness of group processes and unconscious processes that are likely to affect the primary task of the group;

- that they recognize that becoming an accredited Balint leader is a not an end but a beginning.

6. Leaders should receive adequate and continuing supervision.

* to be determined by accrediting societies

** may not be possible at present in some societies

www.balintinternational.com

Criteria for the Accreditation of Balint Group Leaders in Germany

The following prerequisites must be met for <u>medical doctors</u>:

Membership of the German Balint Society, the latest being after the first Leaders' Seminar;

1. Payment of 100,-€ Registration fee when starting the Leaders' Training;

2. Additional training in Psychotherapy or Psychoanalysis or specialization in Psychotherapeutic Medicine or Psychosomatics or Psychiatry and Psychotherapy or in Child and Youth Psychiatry and Psychotherapy;

3. After having finished the above mentioned training, three years of professional work in these fields. During these 3 years you have to be a member of a Balint group either in a continuous

group lead by a group leader who has been accredited by the German Balint Society or at weekend workshops carried out by the German Balint Society for at least 70 Balint Group Sessions;

4. If you did not attend Balint Group Sessions during your additional training or specialization as mentioned in 3. you have to be a member of a continuous Balint Group for another 35 Sessions lead by a Balint Group Leader accredited by the German Balint Society;

5. Participation in six Balint Leaders' Seminars with at least 30 sessions facilitated by a trainer accredited by the German Balint Society. At least four of these Seminars have to be at workshops of the German Balint Society. During the Leaders' Seminars you have to lead at least two group sessions under supervision;

6. Experience in Co-Leading in a continuous group or at workshops of the German Balint Society is required;

7. Accreditation is decided by the Board of the German Balint Society together with the Training Committee;

8. Completing and sending in the application form, which you find on our homepage: *www.balintgesellschaft.de*

The following prerequisites must be met for <u>psychologists</u>:

1. Accredited Psychologists with an additional training in Psychotherapy or Psychoanalysis;

2. After finishing the additional training three years of professional work in Psychotherapy or Psychoanalysis;

3. 105 (one hundred and five) Sessions of Balint Group work lead by a Balint Group Leader accredited by the German Balint Society;

4. At least 35 of these sessions in a continuous group;

5. Participation in six Balint Leaders' Seminars with at least 30 sessions facilitated by a trainer accredited by the German Balint Society. At least four of these Seminars have to be at workshops of the German Balint Society. During the Leaders' Seminars you have to lead at least two group sessions under supervision;

6. Membership of the German Balint Society, the latest being after the first Leaders' Seminar;

7. Experience in Co-Leading in a continuous group or at workshops of the German Balint Society is required;

8. Accreditation is decided by the Board of the German Balint Society together with the Training Committee;

9. Payment of 100,-€ Accreditation fee;

10. Completing and sending in the application form which you find on our homepage: *www.balintgesellschaft.de*

带领巴林特小组指南

LEADING A BALINT GROUP

原著　[德]海德·奥登

主审　魏　镜

主译　史丽丽

中华医学电子音像出版社

CHINESE MEDICAL MULTIMEDIA PRESS

北　京

图书在版编目（CIP）数据

带领巴林特小组指南：英汉对照 /（德）海德·奥登著；史丽丽译. —北京：中华医学电子音像出版社，2021.05

ISBN 978-7-83005-315-4

Ⅰ．①带…　Ⅱ．①海…②史…　Ⅲ．①医院 - 人间关系 - 指南 - 英、汉　Ⅳ．① R197.322-62

中国版本图书馆 CIP 数据核字（2021）第 017778 号

版权登记号　01-2020-0164

Otten, Heide: Leading a Balint group.A guide © PSYLLABUS Publishing House, 2017
The translation was undertaken by Chinese Medical Multimedia Press Co., Ltd. This edition of"Leading a Balint group.Aguide" by Heide Otten is published by arrangement with PSYLLABUS Publishing House.This book is a mutual project of Dr. Heide Otten and PSYLLABUS Publishing House.

带领巴林特小组指南
DAILING BALINTE XIAOZU ZHINAN

主　　译：史丽丽
策划编辑：史仲静
责任编辑：崔竹青青
校　　对：张　娟
责任印刷：李振坤
出版发行：中华医学电子音像出版社
通信地址：北京市西城区东河沿街 69 号中华医学会 610 室
邮　　编：100052
E - mail：cma-cmc@cma.org.cn
购书热线：010-51322675
经　　销：新华书店
印　　刷：廊坊市祥丰印刷有限公司
开　　本：880 mm×1230　mm　1/32
印　　张：5.5
字　　数：150 千字
版　　次：2021 年 5 月第 1 版　　2021 年 5 月第 1 次印刷
定　　价：58.00 元

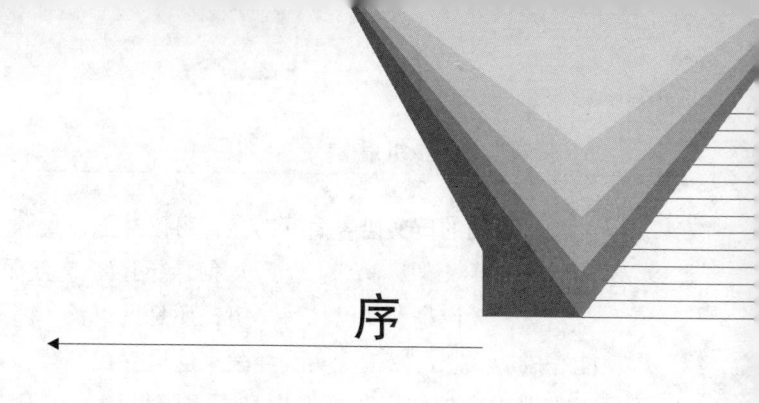

序

    十余年来，随着巴林特小组这种职业化医患关系的工作形式进入更多中国医务工作者的视野，越来越多医务工作者带来自己的医患关系案例，在小组中释放情绪，得到支持，听取反馈，拓宽视野，深入反思……

    有兴趣的人或许会问"我在哪里可以找到一个巴林特小组？"

    有需求的机构或团队问"我们如何引入一个巴林特组长？"

    很多同行在第一次参加或者观摩巴林特小组后，问"怎样才能成为一名巴林特小组的组长？"

    中国巴林特联盟从2012年开始，组织严格的组长培训，由国际巴林特联盟资深专家授课和督导。至2019年参照国际惯例和标准，进行了首次组长认证。Heide Otten 医生是国际巴林特联盟的前主席和经验丰富的组长培训师，一直热心参与中国的巴林特小组工作和组长培训，从2012年首次组长培训到2019年首次组长认证都有她的指导和贡献。

    本书聚焦于巴林特小组的组长功能和培训成长，以清晰的框架介绍了巴林特小组的基本概念流程、组长需要掌握的知识和技能，以及如何形成个性化的组长风格、如何培训组长等重要议题。使用丰富的巴林特小组案例，帮助读者理解小组动力和组长的干预，并从 Otten 医生本人的专家视角分析案例中组长的成败。无论是巴林特小组的入门级组长，还是有经验的组长们，都能在书中发现自己所需要的内容。

作者使用的英文语言简练易懂，可读性强，我们将之翻译成中文，形成中英双语版本，有助于读者对照阅读，方便而不失其原味。

当然，无论是参加巴林特小组，还是做组长，都不是通过阅读就能完成的。您可以带着实践经验来这里寻找答案、验证想法，也可以带着书中的知识和观点投身于组长培训并在工作中带组。实践－总结－再实践－再总结……这既是本书作者输出智慧结晶的方式，也是每一位组长工作和成长的必经之路。

感谢 Heide Otten 医生和所有为中国巴林特工作付出努力的专家们！

魏 镜

2021 年 3 月 25 日，北京

目　录

01 米歇尔·巴林特是谁

1896 年 12 月 3 日，米歇尔·巴林特（Michael Balint，1896—1970 年）出生于匈牙利的布达佩斯。他的父亲在布达佩斯做家庭医生。巴林特同样学医，他对医学和精神分析学都很感兴趣。精神分析由西格蒙德·弗洛伊德（Sigmund Freud，1856—1939 年）和维亚纳的约瑟夫·布洛伊尔（Josef Breuer，1842—1925 年）开创发展，他们也是精神分析学派的代表人物。巴林特阅读弗洛伊德的著作后，非常认同其思想。在职业生涯的早期，巴林特即对心身疾病很感兴趣，重视医疗中的心理学观点。他的理念是让家庭医生具备敏感性，体验到除躯体因素外，心理因素在疾病的发生、发展中也扮演了重要的角色。他和伦敦的同事以小组形式讨论这些问题，并将小组命名为"关系培训暨研究小组"。

在柏林沃博格生化研究所，巴林特在对药物的作用和不良反应进行科学研究的过程中，进一步发展了医生对患者及其疾病影响的理论。他的观点是，医生本身像药物一样发生着作用，包括治疗作用和不良反应。医生与患者交谈的方式、开取药物的方式都会影响患者的康复。他希望通过全科医生小组的研究发现这一规律。在巴林特的著作《医生，他的患者及所患疾病》（巴林特，1957 年）中，他报道了相关研究结果。

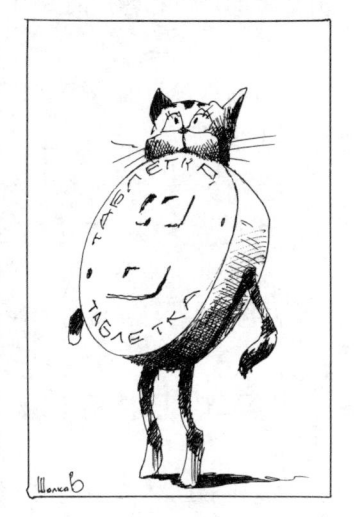

医生是一味药

02 巴林特小组是什么

第二次世界大战后，巴林特开始在伦敦的家庭医生中开展巴林特小组工作。当时，家庭医生接诊一些经历战争创伤的患者，他们有心身疾病的症状，而医生很难理解和处理这些，他们要求接受巴林特的培训。

巴林特对小组成员进行心身思维训练，同时对"医生药物"的治疗作用、医患关系对诊断治疗的影响进行研究。

时至今日，巴林特小组用于训练助人行业的从业者，帮助他们理解职业关系中的困难，从业者从中获得宽慰，避免职业耗竭，提升患者的预后和客户的能力。

目前，参与巴林特小组正式的既定目标包括：
① 提高反思；
② 认识助人者－患者关系的重要性；
③ 提高应对情绪的能力；
④ 感知与观察沟通方式的影响；
⑤ 了解医患互动的治疗作用和不理想的负面作用。

"经典"巴林特小组

经典的巴林特小组由 8～12 位组员组成，有 1 位或 2 位组长。由 1 位组员提供 1 个案例，他讲述患者（客户）的故事，寻求小组

帮助他发现这段职业关系中发生了什么。案例提供者不需要任何记录，他应当自由地叙述，提到哪些内容、遗漏哪些内容，这也是有趣的发现。案例讲述者报告案例的过程中不应被打断，报告过程会表现他的心境和情绪。随后组员在事实层面对案例提出澄清性问题，但也许没有人提问，也许会出现很多重要的问题。这个步骤可能已经是平行进程的一部分了，我们之后再讨论。提问结束后，组长请案例提供者后退一些，接下去的一段时间他将不间断地倾听组员讨论，这有机会注意到对案例的反馈及自己的情绪。如果他保持对小组工作的关注，他可能会感到有义务去更正信息或回答更多问题，也可能想为自己或患者辩护。当后退时，案例提供者仿佛处于患者的位置，不能参与医生的思考、分享医生的感受，这也支持了平行进程，案例提供者可以了解小组中被其案例所激发和表达出的情绪。当案例提供者被请回小组后，他可能会表达自己的感受，或者补充一些想到的可能很重要的内容。组长可以请案例提供者继续倾听小组就新信息展开的讨论。在小组讨论结束之前，案例提供者回到小组之中，再次表述自己的想法、变化和情绪。

这是分析性的小组设置。参与者应用自由联想、想象、画面、猜想和想法等进行工作。巴林特邀请组员们"自由去想""有犯傻的勇气"，既不要使用笔记，也不要学习、引用文献，而是"尽一己之所能"（巴林特，1957年）。案例提供者可以选择哪些评论对自己有用。有时再次见到患者时，他会突然想起一句评论，有恍然大悟之感。

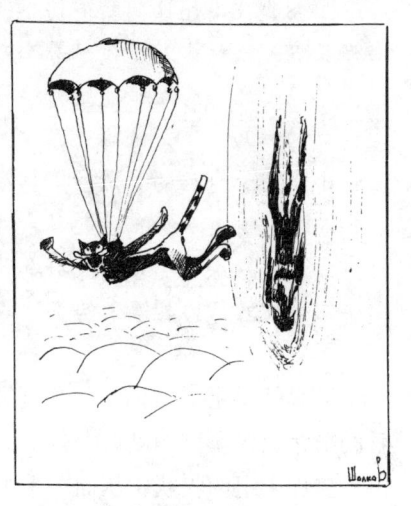

有犯傻的勇气

▶ 案例1：一位年轻家庭医生的案例

　　一位54岁女性患者，首次就诊时由34岁的儿子伴诊。她几乎不能走路，有严重的腹痛。仔细查体和询问病史后，医生决定将患者转诊至妇科做进一步检查，检查结果是宫颈癌。患者的母亲因宫颈癌去世。后续治疗过程中，患者很快中断了放疗、化疗，回到家里。家庭医生尝试说服患者继续接受治疗，但被患者拒绝。最后家庭医生做患者家访。患者有8个子女，最小的女儿13岁。家庭医生对患者提供心理陪伴。患者的一个女儿嫁到巴基斯坦，离婚后回国，但不得不把4个孩子留在巴基斯坦。她感到抑郁，有一次自杀未遂。家庭医生也为她提供了心理支持。患者看中了一家临终关怀机构，要求家庭医生一直陪伴她，医生同意了，但她感到很愤怒：为什么她没有早点来治疗，否则她可以比现在过得更好，她的癌症本来是可以成功治疗的。为什么患者不好好照顾自己？她为家庭付出了一辈子，8个孩子，殚精竭虑的工作……

　　初期，小组认同案例提供者的表现。有位组员强调她十分佩服案例提供者对这位患者和患者家庭的服务，非常重视并付出了很大的努力。她能坚持这样工作多久？她对所有患者都是这样的吗？是不是做得太多了？突然案例提供者热泪盈眶，她被小组给予自己的肯定所震撼了，同时她也意识到，她的表现就像这位有着8个孩子的母亲一样：为别人付出了太多，但对自己关注得太少。她为没有及时注意这一点而感到难过，感谢小组为她的行为和未来的工作打开了天窗。

　　巴林特小组的目标不是找到解决方案，而是为案例提供者和患者的情绪提供不同角度的、新的思路、观点和想法，这也是案例提供者参加小组的收获，从而关系中潜意识的内容进入了意识。

有附加元素的巴林特小组

巴林特在英国伦敦与家庭医生组建第一个小组时，心理治疗理论及实践也继续变化、发展。除了弗洛伊德的"话疗"之外，我们也在个体或团体心理治疗中使用多种创新性的技术，例如：角色扮演、心理剧、雕塑和想象。这些创新性的元素帮助我们识别情绪，让潜意识内容意识化。

在角色扮演中，我们扮演或重演一个情景、一段对话，它们在实际咨询过程中发生过或可能发生。当案例提供者设身处地体会患者的角色，他感受到言语的力量，在真实场景中他对患者使用过或可能使用这些言语。不同的组员可以继续进行角色扮演，我们能感受到细节和差异，清楚地觉察移情和反移情的内涵。更换角色有助于增进理解、促进共情。

> ### 案例2：1个可以展示角色扮演对理解医患互动情景作用的案例

珍妮，一位年轻的家庭医生，在治疗一位76岁依从性欠佳的患者时感到自己无助、无能。患者有严重的背部疼痛，特别是颈部。他经常不预约就临时就诊，而不在预约好的时间就诊，也没有按照之前和家庭医生协商好的那样去看专科医生。他总是带着自己被诊断为痴呆的妻子，声称不能将她独自留在家中，这也是他不去专科进一步就诊的原因。小组对医生表达了共情，她想帮助患者却帮助不到。他们感到沮丧、无助、愤怒。一位组员认同患者的感受，谈到他的负担、孤独和哀伤。衰老并不容易，而现如今家庭越来越小，我们很难再像大家庭那样分配任务和获得支持，几乎所有人都认识像患者这样的人。

案例提供者认真倾听小组的讨论。当回到小组后，她感谢小组对她的理解和支持，但她仍然感到无力，希望将患者转诊至专科诊所，让患者获得治疗，但也确信患者不会接受这个提议，而她会因此感到愤怒。

组长提出进行角色扮演。珍妮扮演了患者，小组中的一位女性精神科医生扮演了珍妮的角色，即家庭医生。

"患者"进入诊室，驼背，颈部僵直，面容痛苦，坐下后就开始抱怨。"医生"平静地应对、倾听，"我理解""这样啊""这个处境很困难""你一辈子都在努力工作，泥瓦匠工作很辛苦。休息是你应得的""有一些诊所可以同时接受你们两位，你和你的妻子。可能她的痴呆也需要治疗。同时你的疼痛也能得到有效缓解，诊所会好好照顾你们两位。""患者"回答："好，我会考虑一下……但你现在能不能给我开点止痛药？""医生"说："好的，我们开一些药物。"等等。

珍妮感到震撼。她感觉自己身体的紧张和疼痛，特别是颈部，同时还有肩部的重压感。她还吃惊地发现，当医生只是共情地倾听，而不是试图说服她时，她的感受多么好。"家庭医生"给了个建议，不多不少，也不给压力，只是让患者想一想。她没有感到难堪，对于家庭医生的建议也没有抵触情绪。有人关爱她，这感觉很温暖。

"我很期待下次咨询。这位患者下周五有一次预约，我希望他会来！"珍妮兴奋地说。

角色扮演使得变换视角更为简单、有效。

心理剧是延伸的角色扮演，由莫雷诺（Moreno）开创。巴林特小组工作与莫雷诺从即兴表演中获得创新的理念完美融合。莫雷诺的自发性概念也解释了巴林特小组中的动力："自发性促进每个人对旧的情境产生新的反应"（Moreno，1974年）。"关系发生变

化的前提是发展出以某种方式去行动的卓越素质，这对于打破常规是必要的。自发的人表现得就像他是新手。每个时刻都是新的"（Krüger，1997 年），这和巴林特"自由去想"的理念也是一致的。他期待小组成员进入情境，感受当时的感受，完全集中于所呈现的故事。

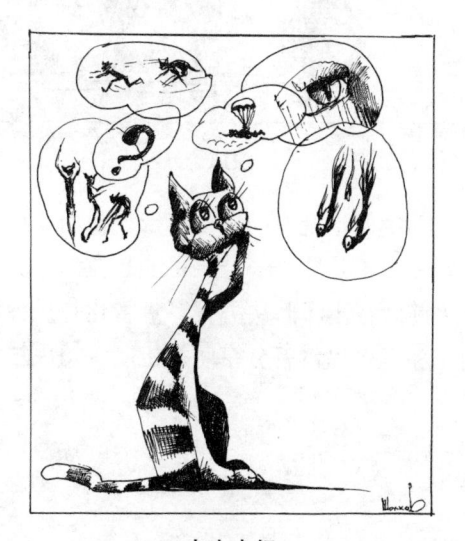

自由去想

创作模拟是一种系统性的方法。这一方法源自 20 世纪 70 年代弗吉尼亚·萨提尔（Virginia Satir，1916—1988 年）创立的家庭治疗。80 年代，希亚·舍恩菲尔德（Thea Schönfelder，1925—2010 年）在吕贝克市举办的"德国北部心理治疗会议"上对这一方法的展示令人印象深刻。小组成员代表问题关系中涉及的"人物"，作为模拟的一部分，案例提供者有机会在一定距离之外观察由别人代表他所提出的问题。这一距离有助于帮助案例提供者更清晰地观察，发现自己的盲点，获得新的观点，但情感与情绪的性质会发生改变。肢体语言是有效的要素。

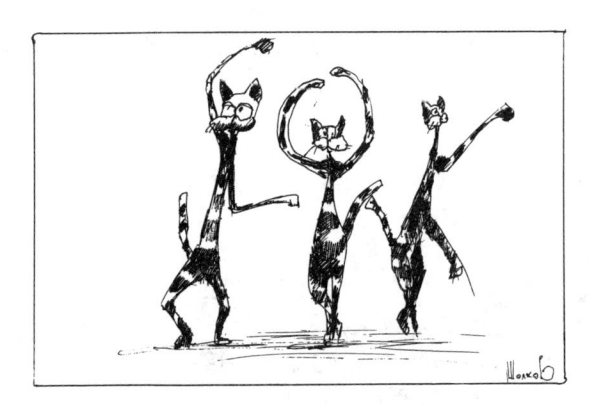

模拟

　　想象技术帮助我们把现有问题变得形象化而非理智化。我们倾向于"想"问题，而不是感受。结果可能是在没有真正理解人物之间发生了什么之前就找出了解决方案，理智化是一种防御机制，有时小组会倾向于和案例提供者分享防御机制，想象技术帮助我们获取新的思路。

> ## 案例 3

　　Christiane 是一位在乡村工作的家庭医生。和其他乡村医生一样，她接诊各个年龄段的患者。一位 16 岁的女孩和母亲一起来就诊，女孩很无礼地要求转诊至两个专科。Christiane 询问她为什么要转诊，女孩的回答更加放肆无礼。最终女孩很不情愿地给医生展示了一小块有些干燥的皮肤，显然不需要转诊至皮肤科。Christiane 给她开了处方，也对她的另一个问题做出了解释：女孩有雷诺病，她的手指有时会变白。女孩在网上了解了和雷诺病相关的知识，要求转诊至专科继续检查。Christiane 解释说，这样做不合适，并与患者预约 1 周后复诊。女孩和母亲一起回来复诊，说上回开的乳霜不管用，不过她的皮肤已经好一些了。女孩的母亲一言不发。Christiane 感到伤

心、被羞辱和愤怒，"如果她是我的女儿，我会好好教育她。她必须尊敬一个成年人、一个医生，不可以有那样的举止。她应该学习礼仪，这个被宠坏的女孩！太没家教了！"

小组成员完全同意。现在的年轻人，部分人的举止不文明，学校里，公共场合等，大多数评论都以"我认为……"或"我会……"开头。

组长请组员们暂停一下，闭上眼睛，任由想象扩展。6分钟后，组长请组员们深呼吸、睁开眼睛，回到小组中谈谈他们看到的图像：一个穿粉色裙子的小公主，一个不停用脚踩地的3岁小孩，她在哭，没人理她，她哭得更凶了，妈妈给了她一块糖就走了。派对上一个时髦的青春期女孩，想表现得很酷、傲慢、高人一等，隐藏内心的不确定、沮丧、反感、孤独等。一个女孩站在大镜子前，看着自己的脸、身体、皮肤，她不满意自己所看到的，而她的母亲则喊着："你看上去太美了！"，这听起来很假，"你撒谎，你根本都没看我！"……一个母亲竖起大拇指："表现好点！"她两手分别拉着一个穿着整齐的小孩边走边说："鸭子一家过马路，妈妈打头，三只小鸭子排在后面……"

在想象环节之后，小组的氛围发生了改变。女孩真正的问题是什么？她到底想表达什么？她为什么要看家庭医生？她为什么要带母亲一起来？医生为什么沮丧？Christiane的愤怒消失了。她吃惊地发现自己几乎忘记了诊室里的母亲。现在她明白母亲也是很重要的，她是对这位母亲感到愤怒，这位母亲没有教育好自己的女儿，没有好好约束她。她也意识到，在年轻女孩表面的傲慢、无礼背后，还有一个不确定、不满足的孩子，她的需求被遮掩了，她自己从未体会到，也未被他人注意。"作为她的家庭医生，我想多了解这个女孩一些。"最后，Christiane这样总结。

想象技术帮助我们进入情绪层面，中止有关道德和政策的讨论，撇开偏见，探询表象以下的深层内容，触及傲慢和无礼行为背后的情绪。案例提供者理解了当时自己一门心思考虑如何比这位母亲更好地教育患者，而没有去分析女孩这种方式背后实际在要求他人真正关注自己的目的。

一些巴林特学者对此持怀疑态度，询问"这还是巴林特小组吗？"。巴林特本人对当时的新治疗技术很感兴趣，例如焦点治疗，在他的培训暨研究小组中加入新的治疗技术也会引起他的兴趣。

如要在巴林特工作中加入以上附加元素，组长应具备特别的知识。我们之后再讨论这一内容。

"金鱼缸"小组

巴林特受邀参与 Sils Maria 在瑞士举办的周末工作坊，他惊讶地发现参加者人数是如此之多。他一直在最多 10 人的小组中开展工作，而当时有 30 位参加者在等他。他们都想体验由巴林特本人带领的小组。他不得不找新的解决方案，也就是我们现在称为"金鱼缸"形式的小组。8～12 位组员构成工作小组，坐成一圈，周围环绕其他参加者。据我所知，巴林特的设计是外圈参加者只能观摩小组进程。时至今日，我们还在一些大型会议中用"金鱼缸"形式做巴林特小组的展示。

如今，外圈成员也可以加入到小组进程中。这些参加者在更远的距离倾听案例，他们可能被引发不同的情绪、联想、幻想。他们倾听内圈小组成员讨论时可能有不同的感受，所以，在小组进程中，组长可基于此邀请外圈成员表达他们的想法和感受，丰富内圈小组的工作。

▶ **案例 4**

在巴林特小组周末工作坊中，参加者自愿组成内圈小组。这个内圈小组中有 8 位组员，24 位参加者坐在外圈。小组中包括家庭医生、精神科医生、妇科医生和儿科医生。组长说明安排后，内圈小组按正常巴林特小组流程工作，外圈成员主要负责倾听，如果组长感到他们可能对内圈小组有帮助，他会邀请外圈成员发表意见、讨论印象。

一位家庭医生提供了案例：他是家乡小镇上的家庭医生，此前父亲也在同一诊所工作。他认识镇上的大部分人，现在他们成了他的患者，有时这会让他的工作和医患关系变得困难。这次他想讨论一位患者，是他的同学，也是他的邻居，他们的妻子和孩子都是好朋友。去年，这个男人患了双相情感障碍，住院治疗 3 个月，出院后回到镇上，希望获得朋友的照护。起初一切都很顺利，直到患者停止服药。他很快出现躁狂发作，想亲近家庭医生的妻子，遭到了她的拒绝，他很生气，把她拽到阳台上，想推她下去。医生非常不安，一方面对此行为极其愤怒，另一方面他又不忍心自己的朋友独自面对这一困难处境。因为患者的严重疾病，他感到无助，也对此感到无望。

首先小组成员延续了他的愤怒，然后是他的担心和无助感。一些女性组员认同他的妻子，她过得不容易，当然应该确信丈夫能保护她。一些成员了解他的矛盾，两家人关系很亲近而不只是邻居而已。一段时间后，小组工作仿佛陷入了无效循环。组长意识到这一点后，决定询问外圈成员的印象。小组之外参加者的情绪没有那么激烈。他们认可矛盾、愤怒、恐惧的体验，但对这一情景有更职业化、更深层次的观点。他们讨论角色的混乱：朋友、家庭医生、精神科医生、社工等，全部角色集于一身。这太多了，负担太重，想找到能分担负担的人。

内圈小组感到释然。现在他们能想象不同的设置，案例提供者也感到释然。他感到可以自由地和其他专业人士合作，请其他做家庭医生的同事来照护朋友一家。他决定只当一个好朋友，彼此的关系不亲密也不疏远。

"金鱼缸"形式的小组提供了从更远的距离获得反馈的机会。或许小组本身也能在后续讨论中谈到这些内容，组长也可以做出相应的干预，但是为什么不借用外界的观察呢？

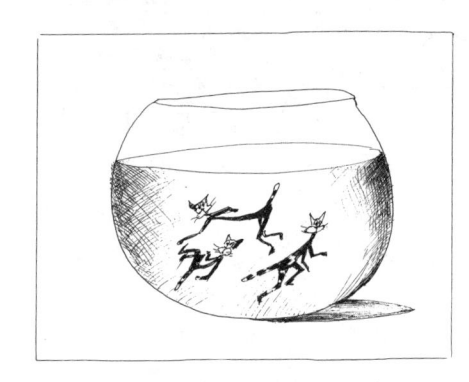

金鱼缸

"金鱼缸"形式的小组通常用于大型会议或周末工作坊，参与人数可以超过小组人数。

组长研讨会

"金鱼缸"形式的小组设置也用于组长研讨会。理想情况下，组长培训中的巴林特小组应有 15 名参加者。我们后面再讨论参加组长培训的要求。

在组长研讨会中，每个人都有机会体验不同的组内角色，这有助于我们理解巴林特小组的进程。所以，在培训中，我们要作为组员、案例提供者、组长或副组长，也要坐在小组外作为观察者探询小组动力、进程、平行进程，以及组长的干预和行为对小组工作、组员及案例提供者的影响。

① 作为小组成员：你的体验如何？组长好好关照你了吗？他们保护你了吗？你有想说的话但没机会表达时，他们注意到了吗？你能自由叙述、表达情绪、自由去想，或说一些"犯傻"的话吗？就像巴林特表达的那样——"有犯傻的勇气"？

运用不被理性和质疑筛选的自由联想是很重要的。所有的发言都像鲜花——案例提供者不但可以把整束花带回家，香味留存在记忆中，当他再次和患者见面，还会记得鲜花的香味。

组长有没有尊重你的发言，他们有没有重视你的想法？

组长对不同想法和贡献的重要性排序是有影响力的，因为当他强调或重复一位组员的发言时，发言内容给人的印象会更深刻。

如果你表达了不适，组长能接受吗？也许之后将其作为案例

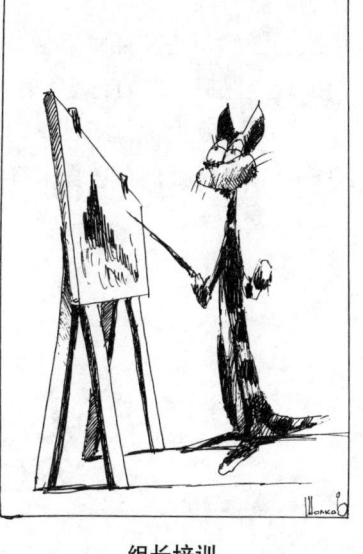

组长培训

动力的一部分做了解释？如果他接受了，那么每个组员都能自由地表达愤怒、不满、嫉妒，以及所有我们认为作为专业人士不应有的情绪。

② 作为案例提供者：感觉如何？在小组中感到安全吗？特别是当组长请你后退、倾听小组就你的医患关系进行讨论时，讲述你的故事而又不能影响小组进程，这需要很多信任。组长和案例提供者保持接触是很重要的，确保小组没有遗弃后退的案例提供者。如有需要，会请案例提供者回到小组中。当有组员反对或贬低你的工作时，组长必须做出反应。你记得他们如何支持一些观点，又弱化了一些观点吗？组长的有趣任务之一是发现平行进程，并让小组成员都看到它。我们之后会讨论这一重要话题。

③ 作为观察者：参与巴林特小组的进程，但坐在小组之外，观察小组中发生了什么。

在这个位置，你应跟随小组动力。你观察组长的干预造成什么

影响。有时你可以猜到组长对关系的假设是什么，看到他尝试说服小组，强调一些发言而忽略另一些发言。你也可能注意到组长对不同的观点保持开放的态度，他可以从新的角度开始考虑。

你可以观察两位组长，他们如何共同工作，如何分配任务，竞争或是互补。他们在进程中有不同角色，是移情和反移情的客体。

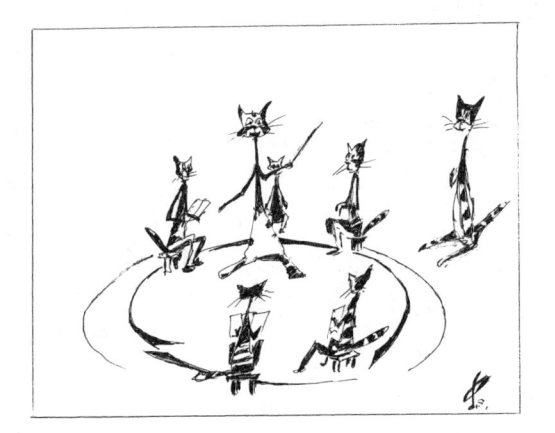

后退

④ 作为组长之一：你感受到自己的不确定性吗？第一次担任这个角色是什么感觉？你可以依赖副组长吗？

对案例提供者、组员、小组进程、平行进程……乃至对你自己的情绪都保持关注，这并不容易。

组长工作听起来比较累，这确实是一个挑战，但也会有一些让人受益的方面。

作为组长的好处就是在小组工作时，你可以反观自身。为处理一段关系，我们通常用 90 分钟进行小组工作。这使得仔细、放松地倾听案例提供者的故事和小组发言成为可能。在倾听时，你可以反观自己针对案例或小组进程的移情或反移情。

小组成员提问时，例如澄清性问题，组长注意到哪些问题有人

问，哪些问题没有人问。为什么没有人想知道患者有没有家人？为什么没有人问到他的社会生活、性功能、工作？你记住这些，如果之后没有小组成员提到相关内容，你就可以提出这一点。因为也许这些内容是有意义的。

　　小组开始工作后，你作为组长，可以暂时注意自己的情绪，探询对关系的假设。同时倾听小组成员的发言，观察案例提供者的反应。

　　如果案例引发了作为组长的你的强烈情绪，那么能有一个副组长辅助是非常重要的，副组长观察到你的情绪，可以替你引导小组进程，直到你能够回到组长的位置。

　　作为组长，你在情绪和元位置（注：元位置是心理治疗领域的术语，是指高于平常的视角，以这个视角可以更客观反思，也有人比喻其为"第三只眼"）之间。这样一来，你就可以与自己的情绪、思维、记忆、经历、移情与反移情、副组长、案例提供者、小组及案例保持联系。

　　就像心理治疗中我们的移情和反移情一样，作为巴林特小组组长，我们的共情和情绪反应也是工具。医生"必须学习如何熟练使用工具，就像外科医生使用手术刀、内科医生使用听诊器、放射科医生使用灯箱一样"（巴林特，1957 年）。

　　因此，在开始组长培训之前，自我体验培训是必需的。

　　我们是和小组一起工作，因此，有关团体动力学的知识也是必需的。

　　巴林特小组的设置是有效和独具特色的，与其他小组设置不同。小组动力非常重要，往往与案例形成镜像，这也是我们在巴林特小组工作中重要的工具。

　　在组长培训中，我们通常用 45 分钟进行小组工作，另外 45 分钟从不同角色的角度讨论小组进程：小组成员感受如何？观察者观察到了什么？案例提供者感到安全吗？他从小组进程中获得了什

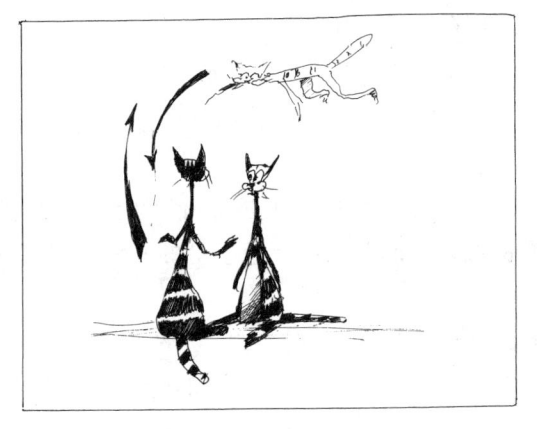

在情绪和元位置之间来回

么？组长的目标是什么？他们对医患关系中的困境有何假设？他们支持新的思路吗？他们在自己的角色中感到舒适、确定吗？组长提到平行进程了吗？组长对小组进程有何影响？案例提供者的收获源自什么？

03 巴林特小组不是什么

案例讨论小组

提起巴林特小组，我们应记住：它需要的是幻想、自由联想、情绪表达、对医患关系的关注。

在案例讨论小组中，首先我们要理智地关注诊断和治疗。我们想知道体格检查、血液学检测、X线片、磁共振等所有结果。在精神科的案例中，我们当然也会关注移情和反移情，因为它们是我们诊断的工具。我们参考患者的病历资料，对治疗的讨论应基于所有的诊断发现更多在理智层面讨论而不是情感层面。

治疗团体

治疗团体的组长是一位专业人士，而团员则是患者。组长利用团体动力学、移情和反移情治疗团体中的患者。被防御的情绪和能量得以在团体中展示，被用于加深理解和治疗康复。团员通过互相交流获得社交训练。他们可以获得针对自己行为的公开反馈，学习应对和解决冲突，处理自己和他人的攻击性行为。团员的社交能力会逐渐成长。团体内的关系是工作重点。团员可以在受保护的环境中获得新的经验。

督导

督导有以下几种不同设置。

① 科室内部团体督导：这种设置可以改善氛围和工作过程。团体和督导师设定目标，首先找出问题在哪里，然后共同寻找解决方案。这些讨论的内容包括实际工作、团体中的不同角色和相互动力。

② 案例督导：聚焦于团体与患者之间的动力。这和巴林特小组工作比较相近。职业人士和客户之间的关系很重要，移情和反移情也被纳入其中。区别在于，我们寻找的是解决方案，我们针对事实层面和组织层面的问题，尝试加以解决。

③ 助人专业人员训练的督导：如精神科医生和心理治疗师，关注的是诊断和治疗。这对受训者来说是必需的。督导的目的在于受训医生治疗患者的全过程，由有经验的同事来监督受训医生的治疗行为。督导组中不应超过4位受训者。这是有效的方法，受训医生可以学习更多的患者实例，他们可以讨论心理治疗技术，彼此学习。这也是案例讨论，而团体动力作为工具不像巴林特小组中那样有必要。

督导有教学的意义，而巴林特小组主要是可以让组员开阔视野、变换视角的。

自我体验团体

在接受心理治疗师培训期间，参加自我体验团体是必需的。我们可以增进对精神动力学、情绪、动机、行为、反应、移情和反移情的了解。

这些都是我们在职业中需要的工具。巴林特说过，医生必须学习如何熟练使用工具，就像外科医生使用手术刀。与团体治疗类似，团体聚焦于团员和他的行为。在开始治疗患者之前，了解自己被防御的情绪和能量是很重要的。我们可以学习和他人换位、更换视角，从而更好地了解自己和患者。

巴林特小组中总是有自我体验的部分。当我们获得小组对医患关系的反馈时，我们更了解自己了。我们谈论和患者的关系，意识到自己的动机和困难之处。小组并不只关注这一点，还可以激发我们更多的自我反思。

自我体验团体更关注我们情绪反应和行为的根源，我们的原生家庭、我们的生活状态、我们深层的情绪，如和伴侣的关系。而巴林特小组，对这部分内容不做讨论，也不做询问。

作为一名巴林特小组组长，自我体验是不可或缺的。当坐在小组中，他必须在情绪和元位置之间来回体验。为了做到这一点，他要意识到自己的情绪和反应，移情和反移情，要区别并处理它们。如果将这些表现出来，可能会破坏小组工作。

小组有自我体验的元素，不只是对案例提供者，也包括所有组员，他们都能在不谈及个人隐私的情况下更了解自己。工作重点不是医生的人格和个人生活，而是医患关系、对患者主诉和症状的了解、医生无意识的回答。

分析医患关系意味着两点：看到患者的冲突、需求、痛苦、疾病，同时看到医生有意识和无意识的回答。

04 巴林特小组的组长要做什么

我在这一领域最重要的老师是沃纳·斯图克（Werner Stucke），他常说的一句话是："作为巴林特小组的组长，你什么都可以做，你不会做错什么，但你要知道自己在做什么。"我想补充一句话："你也要知道自己对案例提供者、案例、组员等的态度，以及你的干预有何影响。"

一方面，组长是小组进程的一部分。他和组员一样倾听案例。他有自己的思想、感受，有对医生、患者和医患关系的假设。

同时，组长也指导着小组进程，观察组员的反应并做出适当干预。他思考怎样将小组进程结构化，以达到允许和给出空间、结构化和限制之间的平衡。不能太多，也不能太少。例如，何时打断案例提供者的报告呢？很多有意义的问题需要提，还是最好直接请组员分享刚才的情绪和反应？问多少个问题？如果问题太多，组长应当打断组员提问吗？如何打断？或者他应该不干预，而是评论"这么多问题意味着什么？"何时引入新的思路、总结，或者点评正在进行的讨论？

组长的决定影响小组进程。结果是什么？这和案例、医患关系有关吗？我们是为案例提供者工作吗？我们还关注他吗？他该离开小组还是回到小组？

倾听小组讨论时，组长有意识地做出决定。他随时注意观察小组的反应。

我们设想一下，如果组长有强烈的假设，并试图让小组跟着他的假设走。那么会发生什么呢？小组可能会跟着组长走，也可能会出现其他情况。如果他没有意识到这一点，仍然和小组对抗，小

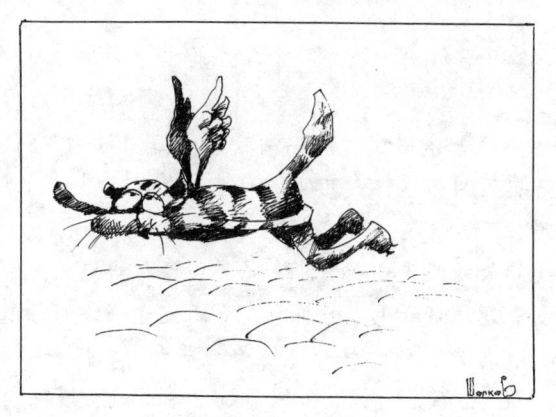

自由悬浮的主意

组的讨论就会无效、勉强、重复。如果他注意到自己和小组的方向不一致，他可以做出评论，继续试图说服小组，也可以跟随组员的思路和表达改变自己的假设，获得新的想法。他带着自由悬浮的主意，用开放的思想跟随小组讨论。

他也会关注案例提供者的安全、反应、何时回归小组讨论，以及小组的主题——医患关系。

> **案例 5**

  一位年轻的家庭医生报告案例。他在父亲的私人诊所工作了半年。父亲希望自己逐步减少工作，让他承担更多任务。于是，他必须照护一对年迈夫妻。父亲告诉他："小心他们，特别是妻子，她可不好对付。15 年之前她还是我们社区的护士，有点专横。"年轻医生第一次做家访，他体会到了父亲告诉他的内容。他和老先生对话，但总是由妻子代为回答。她不想让医生给自己的丈夫查体，而是希望医生开了药就走。年轻医生对此感到不快，医生看到他们的情况并不好，如这位妻子给丈夫服用的临时药物会加重他的病情。他细心地解释，但她不听

医生的。妻子强调自己有多年医学经验，他太年轻不明白。她根本不重视他的意见。他又尝试做了一次家访，然后就放弃了，让她另找一个医生。他感到轻松，但同时又觉得不甘心。他不理解自己为何这样：其实他有很多患者，愿意听他意见的患者都照护不过来。

小组组长的假设是：医生害怕被父亲批评。他觉得自己失败了，没有处理好和患者的关系。带着这个假设，组长强调了小组中所有与此一致的评论。组长可能会说："超越父亲是很困难的。"小组会就这个话题展开讨论。可能会有组员或副组长（如果有）将注意力带回两位患者身上："那位老先生呢？我同情他。他没有机会和医生建立联系，也许医生挺喜欢他的。"这会是一个重要的新视角。

如果组长坚持自己的假设，他很有可能会回到假设上，不给组员更多展开讨论的机会（"如果医生真的喜欢他，为什么不再接诊呢？"），或者谈起诊所的结构（"丢失或抛弃患者是怎么回事？这是不是案例提供者父亲的主题？"）。

一个对新思路、新视角开放的组长会紧接这个话题，"好的，你感到他喜欢老先生。那案例提供者现在怎么看呢？"

另一位组员可能会关注年迈的妻子。她真的傲慢吗？还是焦虑？她想获得控制权吗？她的护士职业生涯让她和医生相处并从中获得了什么经验？

有着强烈假设的组长可能会问："或者她只是对年轻医生感到怀疑，就像他父亲对他那样？父亲真的相信他吗？他能放心依赖儿子，将患者交给他吗？"

保持开放态度的组长可能对这个思路感兴趣并表达支持："这是一个好问题。她真的不信任医生吗？或者她只是想表达自己的焦虑和疑虑？她可能想寻找一位像父亲那样自信的医生，他能让她平静，告诉她紧急情况下应采取哪些正确的方法。"

　　巴林特小组一般不寻求解决方案。小组为案例提供者提供建议、自由联想、思路。案例提供者决定哪些对自己重要，哪些揭示了自己的盲点，哪些给了自己新思路；这一过程可能在小组工作结束后仍会继续，如案例提供者再次见到患者时。组长负责激发并收集组员们的这些提议。在我们的案例中，他对各个角度保持开放的态度：案例提供者与父亲的关系、与患者的关系、与患者妻子的关系，他的不确定，他的理想，他的边界等。

　　倾听案例提供者时，小组里的每个人都会快速建立一个假设。组员首次发言时，我们就能听到这些假设。"自由去想"是巴林特的名言。因为所有的发言都很宝贵，反映了案例提供者的潜意识和意识。处于元位置的组长必须辨别自己的自发假设和对小组有益的评论。

　　小组中有副组长时，组长和副组长要保持联系。小组中有两位组长应当是令人宽慰的，他们可以分担重要的任务和职责。重要的是，组长和副组长都要在专注倾听和元位置之间来回切换，关注小组中发生了什么，两位也都能影响小组进程。

　　我们主要在组长工作坊中训练这一点。

　　这不是对与错、好与坏的问题，而是自我识别和感知的问题。

　　组长曾作为组员，学习如何耐心、仔细地倾听他人发言，尊重他人，使组员们有足够的安全感去想象和"自由去想"，这也是他带领小组的任务。

　　作为小组成员，或被督导的组长、副组长，或在小组外观察工作，这些不同的经历都是培训和学习过程中的重要组成部分。

　　分析小组进程、组长对小组的影响、小组的氛围，这些是组长培训中要做的第二部分工作，一位经历过良好培训的组长在带组时会知晓这些内容，并做出相应的干预。

　　带领巴林特小组可被视为一种技术，只有保持自我感知才能运用自如。

　　盖多·弗莱腾（Guido Flatten）在研究中发现，组员将组长的存在和行为视为对小组工作最重要的影响因素。

　　而巴林特写道："可能最重要的因素就是小组组长的行为。毫不夸张地说，如果组长态度正确，他以身作则就比其他任何因素加起来更具有教育意义。毕竟我们提倡的这种技术，就是基于我们期待医生学到、并用于患者的倾听技巧。允许每个人做自己，让他们有时间表达内心所想，关注合适的节点——也就是，只在真正需要发言时发言，他要表达的不是正确的方法，而是使医生们有可能自己发现并处理患者问题的正确方法——组长可以'当时当地'展示他想要教授的内容。很显然，没有人可以完全达到这些标准。幸运的是，我们并不需要完美。组长可以犯错——实际上组长时常犯错，但这不会造成多少伤害，如果他能接受相当于或更甚于他希望小组所能接受的批评。"（巴林特，1957 年）

　　巴林特指出，组长是一个榜样。他处理小组发言的方式、倾听和接纳并认可新思路的方式，都是小组内互动和医患互动的榜样。就像参加者在巴林特小组中寻求帮助那样，组长出错之后，他也可能寻求副组长的帮助。

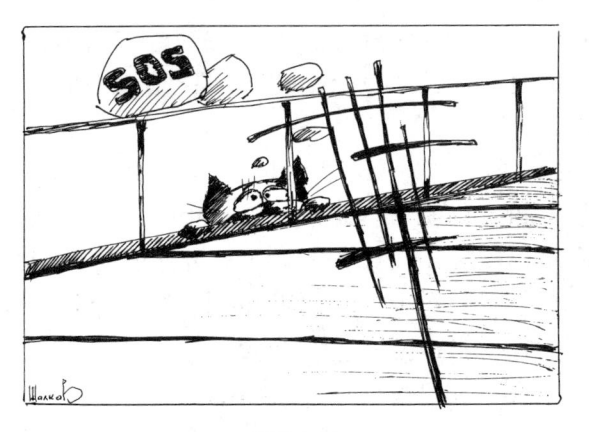

出错之后

伦理假设与限制

组长传达的很重要的信息之一是彼此尊重、认可组员的思想。组员可能来自不同文化的背景，拥有不同宗教信仰和世界观。案例中的患者可能很奇怪，有不正确的行为，要求太多。尊重是很重要的。"为什么"这样的问题总是存在。我们能理解发生了什么吗？

理解和接受当然是有限度的。

"自由去想"并不意味着去伤害、破坏或攻击。组长要辨别能推动反思的评论和过分、无帮助的攻击性评论，这往往如同走钢丝。识别平行进程是很重要的。一位组员对另一位组员的人身攻击是越界行为。组长要指出并阻止这一行为，因为小组的安全性是很重要的。

在巴林特小组中，问题不在于"对或错""不是，就是"，而在于"也"。接受对立的思维和观念、接纳矛盾是重要的。

巴林特小组的成功依赖于组员的诚实、公开、尊重和互相支持。保密原则也是很重要的，小组共同工作的时间越长，小组凝聚力和信任感就会越强。

案例提供者和组员的安全性

组长的责任是在给出空间和结构化之间维持平衡。组员在安全的氛围中自由表达思想、想象、感受时，小组工作丰富、有成效。组长怎样建立这样的氛围呢？保持警觉、注意力集中、积极、友好、确定、严格、清晰、设置边界——这些都是组长的特质，他应保证小组安全、有创意的氛围。放肆的想法可以被允许，笑声也能被接受，只要这些不造成伤害。对这些表达的限制不等于打断它们，而是明确指出它们。组长可以尝试给出一个解释，如他可以提

问："为什么这个时候有了笑声？我们在回避什么情绪吗？""这里的笑声是什么意思，羞耻的，攻击性的，还是贬低性的？"组长总是要留意案例提供者，特别是在其后退之后。组长可以随时请案例提供者回归小组并询问他的感受。

保密原则

　　小组工作开始前，组长应说明小组的任务。他提醒组员要准时，并且小组工作结束前不能离开。如果有人需要临时离开房间，则必须告知原因。保密性是必不可少的原则。小组中的每个人都要确信，组员的发言内容或案例提供者的故事都不会从小组所在的房间泄露。这在临床上尤为重要，特别是当组员相互认识时，他们一起工作、用餐、闲聊。组员们接受这一观点：小组工作结束后彼此不再互相谈论或和别人讨论小组内容是必不可少的。如果组员对保密原则不能确定，没有人会愿意提供案例，小组讨论也会变得理性化而无聊。

　　保密原则是巴林特小组工作中最重要的原则。这也是我们在有科室员工参与的巴林特小组中不接受科室主任的原因之一，因为这样做会影响小组自由、安全的氛围。

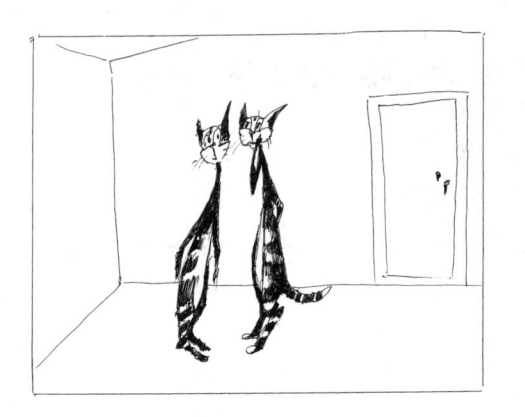

保密原则

解决冲突

巴林特小组中可能出现哪种冲突？组长必须能辨别反映案例内容的冲突和组员之间相处的冲突。如果是平行进程，组长应指出这一点，并带领小组了解并解决冲突。如果是另一种情况，我们从团体动力学中了解到"以扰动为优先"，解决冲突而不是避免冲突，这也是组长的任务之一。组长依然可以作为榜样，如何发现冲突，又如何对待冲突？

在此我想举一个例子。在德国，我们有强制参加的巴林特小组。在培医生必须参加小组，不是每个人都乐意。大部分小组会议都在医生的休息时间举行，如晚上或周末，这使得很多人不情愿参加。在这样一个小组中，有2位成员为细节争斗，诋毁彼此的发言。组长公开说出自己的发现，询问小组成员有何体会。他们抱怨培训中感受到的压力，看似无聊、不必要的强制活动带来的沮丧感，以及日常生活中没有足够时间和家人或朋友相处。小组不需要继续讨论患者，而是需要聊聊他们的个人问题和生活状况。组长提供了这个机会，下一次小组会议，回归到医患关系的讨论。组员们认识到关注医患关系的巴林特小组也关注他们的问题。组长做了示范，也许这些年轻医生会学习到，与抽血化验、体格检查相比，他们更值得花些时间去听患者谈谈困扰。

怎样处理攻击性

攻击性首先是一种能量。我们可以利用它推动事物前进和脱离依赖。巴林特小组中的攻击性可能表现为面对，例如让案例提供者面对自己潜意识中的恐惧、欲望和需求。"自由去想"可能意味着开启攻击性。

"我讨厌这个要求多的患者……""我有一个丑恶的想法，想把他踢出去……"发现攻击冲动和倾向会带来自由和解脱的感觉。仅仅是幻想踢别人一脚，都能让我们笑出来——释怀了。巴林特小组欢迎这样的攻击幻想。

当我们不认可这些幻想，而是将攻击性表现出来时，情况就变得困难了：攻击性可能会表现为贬低、侮辱、冒犯。小组成员甚至可能出现公开争吵。

组长的任务是探究这种现象背后的意义。这是医患关系的一部分吗？充满攻击性的小组反映了案例内容吗？

或者这种攻击动力有其他原因，一个原因可能是小组的强制性，参加者对一直讨论患者已经厌烦了，他们宁愿讨论其他主题或陪伴家人或朋友；另一个原因可能是组员间未知的敌对性，或是其他阶段未解决的冲突。组长要找到原因，也就是公开提出这一点。

组长的自我体验是极其重要的。他学过如何处理攻击性吗？或者攻击性是他家族中的禁忌？或是职业禁忌？人们不会信任一个具有攻击性的医生，因为医生必须永远善良、善解人意、有同情心的。如果组长有类似的理想，接受深层次的情绪会很困难，因为这不符合他的理想。如果组长害怕攻击性情绪而习惯安抚，他可能会失去在巴林特小组中利用攻击性的机会。小组中出现紧张氛围时，他可能会引发更多对攻击性的防御和抑制行为。

针对组长本人的攻击性不容易处理。他需要找出原因，是平行进程吗？反映了案例吗？或是他自己挑起了和小组的争斗？

▶ 案例6

巴林特小组的一些组员显得不安，因为得知新的政策会导致他们的收入下降。他们迫切地希望讨论政策变动，而不是讨论如何处理医患关系。小组组长要求组员等到茶歇时再讨论现

实问题，应立刻开始巴林特工作。一番抗议后，其中一位组员提供了案例。患者是他自己诊所的护士，他的问题在于，她想在手术后请很长时间的病假。他要求她考虑他的财务情况，即他并没有能力请人来替代她的工作。小组赞同他的意见，批评那位患者，并展开了对家庭医生财务情况的讨论。组长做出干预："我的印象是，这个案例有其他重要的方面没有被提及。"这吸引了被他拒绝过的组员们的攻击。

一位有经验的组长会和小组一起分析这个情况："我理解你们生我的气，因为我坚持要讨论医患关系。你们很聪明，这又回到了你们想聊的话题：财务变化。好吧，你们赢了！（微笑）"

在这个案例中，组长并不自信，而小组也是新的要求强制参加的小组。在巴林特小组组长督导中他谈及这一经历。希望他能了解这些内容，下次能尽情地和小组讨论这一点。

05 副组长要做什么

　　巴林特小组有两位组长是有利于开展工作的。他们可以分担如前所述的多项任务。两位组长在小组中相对而坐，以获得不同的视角。一位组长可以观察案例提供者及他的反应，好好照顾他。案例提供者退后，组长必须注意他何时需要回到小组。

　　一位组长通常引导小组进程，另一位组长负责观察。

　　如果案例引发了一位组长强烈的情绪，那么有副组长就很顺利了，因为副组长可以观察到组长的情绪，替他引导小组进程，直到组长能够回归组长角色。

　　合作意识是很重要的。如果两位组长彼此熟识，也共同工作了一段时间，那么他们就可以利用自己的观察。今天他们为什么争斗？这是和案例相关的平行进程吗？他们为什么要竞争？医生和患者在竞争吗？小组尝试让他们分裂吗？这意味着什么？他们是像父母一样，给小组和案例提供者当父亲和母亲吗？这些有助于对小组进程的理解。当两位组长开放性地展示行为并说出他们的立场时，小组成员会感到安全。

支持组长

　　组长的多项任务是可以被分担的。两位组长应在小组工作开始前沟通好分工安排。他们要确定谁负责维系小组结构、给出信息。如果两位组长对案例的思路或带组风格不一致，那么小组工作开展起来并不容易。如果一位组长习惯给组员更多空间，不做过多干预，让小组自由讨论，而副组长习惯结构化的进程，那么明智的

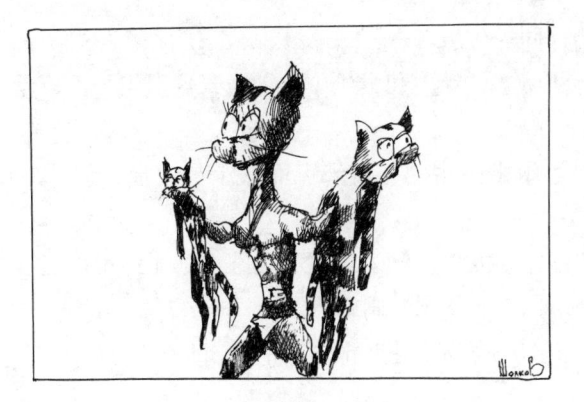

支持

做法是在小组会议开始前讨论这一点并达成一致。一位组长应当主导并带领小组工作。如果两位组长的带组风格有冲突又没有预先解决，小组的工作可能会不顺利。小组会被竞争拖垮，或小组被分裂，进而陷入竞争。两位组长不会给案例提供者和案例足够的空间。设立两位组长的目的是为了互相支持、分担任务，仔细观察小组，为小组成员特别是案例提供者服务。小组工作结束后，两位组长之间进行思路交流也是很有必要的。

反映小组进程

副组长的工作包括仔细观察小组进程，并向小组提供他的反映。

巴林特小组最吸引人的方面是平行进程。我们之后再讨论这一内容。

伯恩·卡里埃尔（Bern Carrière）写过一篇文章："小组动力总是反映案例吗？"

这是一个棘手、困难的问题。

巴林特小组起源于临床工作，组员们除了在巴林特小组中相处之外，还有更多互相接触的机会。他们共同工作、用餐、培训，有

时还会治疗同一位患者。

区分团队中的动力和案例中的动力，这对组长而言是个特殊的挑战。

如果小组由陌生的、素未谋面的组员组成，似乎氛围会轻松一些。

但要注意，我们都知道移情和反移情，小组中可能有组员让我们想起一位同事、父亲、姐妹等。

小组中的所有情绪并非都由案例引发！

照顾组员

两位组长都会关注小组成员。副组长通常有更多时间观察组员，而组长更关注发言、发言者、案例提供者、案例和平行进程。可能有一位安静的组员一直没有发过言。副组长要特别注意这些组员，观察姿势、肢体语言，寻找邀请这位组员加入小组讨论的最佳时机。他可以直接提出要求，也可以指出自己的疑惑，即这位组员为什么沉默。有时这些组员会提到医患关系中非常重要的方面，"我以为没人愿意听我说话""我没什么可说的""我太生气了""我尝试加入讨论，但总有人比我更快一步"或"没必要说什么，大家都说到了"。这位组员可能代表了患者的一部分。小组中的每个组员都代表了患者或案例提供者的一部分。重视并利用这一点是组长的任务。指出小组中的情绪反映了案例中的情绪，这样做可以帮助每一位组员。有时我们能听到这样的发言："我不知道自己怎么了，一般没有这种感受，但在这里我感到被抛弃了，没有力气，逆来顺受，有虐待欲……"

06 平行进程

平行进程是指医患关系的冲突和情绪反映在小组进程中。

通常案例提供者会"置身于"患者的处境，尤其是在后退时。

医生讲述了他与患者的故事，并将这个故事交给了小组，就如同患者把他的故事——主诉及症状，交给了医生。

在不少情况下，患者质疑：医生真的理解了我的意思吗？他得到正确的结论了吗？他真的能帮助我吗？

类似的问题也发生在案例提供者身上：当他向小组报告了案例并后退到小组以外，质疑可能就来了：他能把患者的事情弄清楚吗？他能相信小组，特别是组长吗？他们打算怎么处理自己的问题？他能从中获益吗？

他可能感觉自己像患者一样被照顾得很好，或被抛弃。

在后退的情况下，案例提供者坐在圈外，暂时被小组排除在外——这就像患者在两次就诊之间被排除在医生的照顾以外一样。

在小组工作中，医生和患者的无意识、未被表达的情绪和想法可以被表达或显露出来。

幸运的是，这些想法被"大声地表达"。案例提供者可以看到这个过程，情绪被缓解：患者是不确定的、矛盾的、焦虑的等等

医生也被困住了，他感到无助，无法说服患者，这使他感到愤怒，他被患者惹恼了，他可能再也不想见到患者，另一方面他想向患者提供帮助，但他可能对于诊断和治疗有疑问……

这些都会在小组当中被提到。

有时案例提供者在倾听的过程中已经灵机一动："哦，我们都感到无助、愤怒、矛盾和焦虑……"

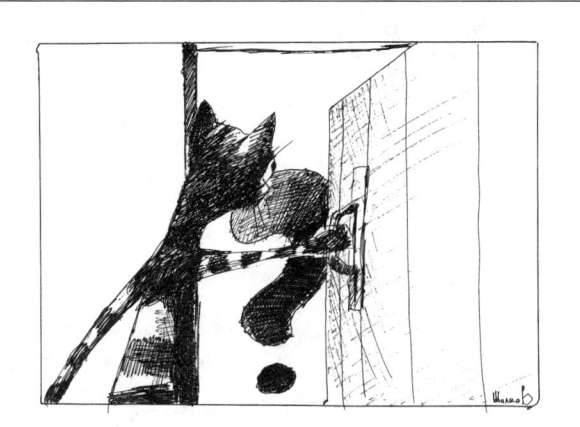

问题还在

　　组长请案例提供者回到小组，他可能会表达他的体会和想法。有时他会补充之前忘了说的重要细节——患者可能在第二次就诊时已经做了类似的事。有时他感到鼓舞或放松，感到被很好地支持，并开始理解了他和患者之间所发生的事。

　　但是，问题可能一直存在。

　　或者案例提供者和之前一样无助。小组工作好像徒劳无功。难道这就是羞辱，是不知感恩，抑或只是平行进程？

　　组长可能让案例提供者再次后退，并观察这个小组，刚才的反馈对他们的工作意味着什么。当他们成功时，感受是什么？当他们看上去失败时，感受又是什么？

　　当然，组长必须关注这些反应，以及对他们的工作意味着什么。组长可能有时在医生的角色中。就好像他面对患者感到沮丧，小组成员和组长也感到沮丧。尽管他们已经很努力地工作，而且这个案例花费了他们很长时间，比医生在患者身上花的时间还多，却还是帮不上忙。

　　理解这种沮丧，并将其放到适当的背景中是很重要的。

▶ 案例 7

一位全科医生告诉小组，她因为一位 42 岁主诉腹痛的女性患者而感到沮丧。4 年前她患了 1 型糖尿病，她父亲和哥哥有 2 型糖尿病。当她在家里抱怨的时候，他们就会反驳说，糖尿病也没什么，他们可以应付，为什么她就不行？

她在一家医疗保险的代理公司工作。同事们不喜欢她在办公桌上测血糖。这让她感到被别人拒绝、批评，甚至不受欢迎。

她向全科医生要求开病假条，全科医生请她再约一次，以便对她的腹痛做进一步检查，患者拒绝了。医生告诉她，如果她不愿听从建议，就不给她开假条，但是全科医生也感觉这样的方式并不好，这看上去像对她的勒索。"我们之间出了什么问题？"

然后，小组对此进行了讨论，小组成员都很努力。组员对医生的无助、愤怒和沮丧表示理解。他们考虑如果换成他们会怎么做，如何说服患者或者迫使她服从，案例提供者回到小组做第一次反馈。小组工作并没有真正帮到她，她没有听到什么新的内容，她想到患者下一次来就诊仍然感到不舒服。

小组成员也感到沮丧。他们认为已经给了很多建议，但这些还是不够。

组长指出这个平行进程，小组和案例提供者都笑了，并且放松下来。这个案例提供者就像是患者，到目前为止小组还没有满足她的需要。

大家继续工作，这次进入了患者的角色。她想要什么，她可能需要什么？"没人能理解，慢性病是多大的负担。"有人从医生的角度说："当 4 年前你得知这个诊断时，对你一定是个打击，而且还很困难。"

> 突然间，案例提供者眼前就像开了一扇门，她不想和患者争吵并迫使她做更多检查，她要做的仅仅是尝试换个角度去想。我们作为医生，看了很多的慢性病患者，但这个患者，因为自己的病被不同的人用不同方式批评和质疑，而她的生命是独一无二的，与父亲和哥哥的不一样。最终，她的医生理解了患者。

在医患关系和巴林特小组－案例提供者之间发生了一个平行进程。

当案例提供者成功地认同了患者及其所有的情绪，从这个角度出发，他能够更好地理解互动关系。

小组工作就像一个放大镜，每一个细节都能被放大，每一种情绪都被描述出来。在日常 5 分钟接诊的时间里所发生的事，现在由 8～12 位专家在 1 个多小时内展开。

在这个过程中，案例提供者处于患者的位置，小组反映出医生的状态，而组长就像是督导者，负责把所有的事情摆到明面上来谈。

07 组长的培训

正如我们所看到的，担任组长的角色需要大量的经验和知识。一个由富有经验的成员所组成的小组也许能自己进行工作。我们的组长培训小组，就能很好地证明这一点。这些组员已经参加过巴林特小组，他们是具有专业经验的心理治疗师，并且了解团体动力。这对组长在小组中的地位以及指导小组工作是个挑战，因为这不同于带领一个新手或学生的小组，也不同于由全科医生或精神科医生或两者均有组成的小组。你的经验越多，做这项工作就能越放松，也能越有趣。你观察了所有的细节并能够使用动力学去帮助案例提供者理解他的困难。

参加组长培训的要求

参加组长培训前你必须完成一些特定的培训。在德国，你必须是医生或临床心理学家并接受心理治疗师的相关培训。

在这个培训中，你必须是自我体验小组成员或者完成了个体的自我体验训练。你已经学习了心理治疗的不同技术，这些在巴林特小组中会用到。而且，你必须作为组员参加过 35 次的巴林特小组。这是参加组长培训的一个重要先决条件。如果你的培训不包含这个内容，必须在巴林特会议或周末工作坊中获取经验。

阶段和标准

国际巴林特联盟的基本要求：

① 组长应该有适当的基础训练，如家庭医生、精神分析师、心理治疗师、心理学家的相关训练。

② 组长应该有参加巴林特小组的经验。

③ 组长应该与有资质的组长一起工作足够长的时间。

④ 组长应该对医患关系有充分的了解。

⑤ 组长应该接受足够的督导。

同时组长应当能够证明具备以下能力：

① 给小组创造安全和自由的环境。

② 工作聚焦于医患关系而非寻求答案。

③ 创造一种学习氛围而非单纯的说教。

在德国我们对组长认证有以下标准：

① 你必须是心理治疗师、精神分析师、心身医学或精神科医生。

② 专业认证后有 3 年的工作经验，另外有参加 70 次巴林特小组的经验。如果在这部分培训中认识不同的有资质的组长更好。

③ 在组长研讨会中接受组长培训。必须参加至少 6 次研讨会，至少接受 30 次小组培训，以获取理论基础和实践经验。

④ 同时，你需要和一个有经验的组长共同带领一个巴林特小组，并担任副组长。

⑤ 心理学家必须有临床培训和附加的作为心理治疗师或精神分析师的教育经历。总共需要作为组员参加 105 次巴林特小组。

经典的巴林特小组

以下是带领一个经典巴林特小组的要求。

经典小组需要精神分析式思维。组长在情绪与理性思维之间，观察和分析之间，此时此地和元位置之间来回切换。平行进程始终在他的头脑中。

组员以他们的共情和认同他人的能力进行工作，这时就可能浮现出各种场景。组长描述情绪并揭示在小组中出现的场景。他的干预是解释小组进程并使之结构化。

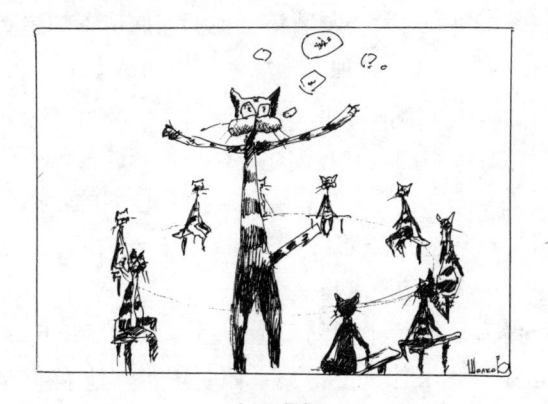

小组进程

带有其他元素的巴林特小组

弗洛伊德把重点放在患者的内在心理冲突上。巴林特考虑到医患之间的互动。今天我们也对系统观感兴趣。

雕塑显示了医生和患者的系统。他们在系统中生活和工作，反过来这些系统影响他们的关系。

让我们想象一下：一位医生，处于不能给患者提供最好治疗的压力之下，因为患者没有足够的钱而医保系统也无法承担。

再想象一位患者，他因为害怕失去工作而不敢休病假。这些因素都会影响医患关系。

你可以让组员们表现这些，让他们代表医生、患者、医保系统、疾病、老板、家庭等。

组长按照常规开始小组工作，案例提供者讲述他的故事，然后进行澄清性提问。

案例提供者选择扮演者并做出模拟，组长会协助他。

当扮演者在他们被指定的位置，案例提供者给他们每人一句话：在这个位置上的想法、感受。

通过片刻的沉默，让扮演者体会他们在此位置的感受，组长问他们："你在这个位置，其他人围绕你，你的感受是什么？""怎么改变这个模拟能让你感觉更好？"

案例提供者仔细倾听，并选择一些角色来改变模拟。可能是一个、两个或更多的人，现在可以尝试去改变他们的状态。案例提供者和其他组员观察这个改变。

然后组长再次采访所有扮演者。

现在已经有了两个不同的模拟画面可以对案例提供者产生影响，忽然间他理解了什么使得关系如此困难。他能够改变他的视角，找出困境的两条出路。

随后的小组讨论这些。

在小组工作中，这个过程添加了什么？

通过使用肢体语言加深了情绪理解。关系和影响因素被视觉化且容易理解。场景的改变可以激活视角。案例提供者更容易后退并达到元位置。

情绪被唤起——尤其是扮演者，也包括观察者——强烈的，留在心里，可以被回忆并改变医患沟通的方式。例如认同患者是一个特殊而重要的情绪体验，同时培养了改变视角的能力。

这种小组动力与分析性设置是不同的。讨论小组可以顺利工作并给场景呈现提供了空间。强烈的思绪被唤起并带回小组讨论和反馈环节。对于所呈现的案例更为专注。模拟工作以后组长回到案例提供者所关心的问题和医患关系。"我们听到了案例提供者的报告，经历了模拟工作。现在你的感受如何？想象和印象是什么？"

通常平行进程被模拟工作强化。

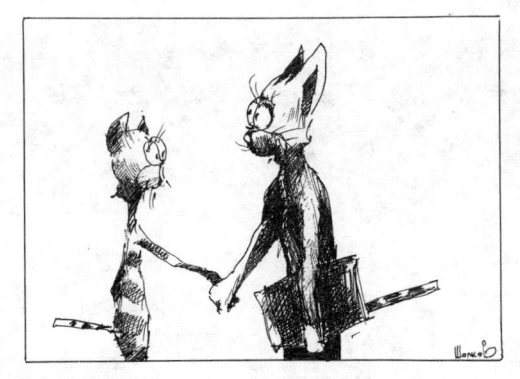

情绪体验

 案例8

　　一个初期的培训中的实习生报告了她在门诊见到的一位患者。他坐在轮椅上被哥哥推进来。患者有神经系统缺陷，医生也不能确定他是否了解了她的病情，因为总是他哥哥回答。哥哥要求必须给患者使用抗生素，因为他尿液混浊。医生在病历中看到，这个患者一发热就用抗生素，而且只用抗生素。她解释说患者过去已经用了太多抗生素，再用没有好处，但是患者哥哥坚持要求。于是她出去请教了一位资深医生，给的建议是先做进一步检查。患者哥哥很生气，但不得不接受。这个情况让她很困扰。

　　在模拟中能感受到空间的狭小和患者哥哥的主观性。令人惊讶的是哥哥的扮演者没有感到这个角色高人一等和苛求，反而是焦虑、不确定和绝望。在第一个模拟中他是唯一站着的人。改变后的模拟3个人都坐着，医生和患者有了目光接触，气氛轻松多了。

　　随后的小组反馈谈到了哥哥，他的态度、感受和行为。组长让这个话题持续了一段时间，然后她说在视野中看不到

案例提供者和患者。案例提供者很感谢这番话。她仔细听着，感觉到她和她关心的问题没有被作为重点，但这是她要求小组处理的问题，而她忽然间理解了患者的处境。在接诊当中她只关注与患者哥哥的冲突，而看不见患者，这正是困扰她的真正原因。

在这个平行进程中，案例提供者体验到了患者的情绪，并在模拟中得到支持。哥哥在模拟中成为主角和充斥了讨论。医患关系被抑制，就如同在诊室中一样。

后退技术强化了这种体验。当案例提供者听着讨论，而不表达自己情绪的时候，她接近了患者的沉默角色，现在她可以感受到他并更加关注他的处境。

使用上述附加元素的组长必须有使用这些技术的经验。系统式治疗的培训包含了大部分的上述技术。

带领这种巴林特小组的准备工作包括接受系统性技术培训和经典巴林特工作培训、参加组长研讨会、带领经典巴林特小组，然后接受带领加入创造性元素巴林特小组的其他培训。这些奠定了坚实的基础，可以在小组中提供不同的方法。

重要的是，让小组和案例提供者有选择。在模拟工作中，案例提供者需要配合并比经典巴林特小组做更多，他就是设计家，这需要的他同意。这些小组中情绪更为强烈。当你在模拟中的某个位置时，你感到痛苦、焦虑、筋疲力尽等。扮演者表达这些情感。小组必须对这样的经历有所准备。

08 巴林特小组组长必须意识到什么

在巴林特小组组长工作坊里，我们会得到启示，什么做错了以及何种行为或干预无助于案例提供者。这是培训中非常重要的一部分。正如巴林特所说："组长可能犯错误——事实上他经常犯错——如果他能够接受批评，甚至接受比他所预料小组所能接受的更为尖锐的批评，并不会带来严重伤害……"（*Balint*，1957 年）

这与 W·Stuckes 的观察相一致："作为巴林特小组组长，你可以做任何事，没有什么是错的，只不过你必须意识到你在做什么。"

这两点就是我们在组长研讨会所培训的。在反馈的部分，培训中的组长听取和接受批评是很重要的，这是培训的本质。学会做意味着下次做得更好，为了意识到发生了什么，你需要来自观察者、案例提供者和组员的反馈。到那时，组长就学习到他在小组进程中的干预效果如何，这就是培训的目标。

在经典巴林特小组中

▶ 案例 9

一个年轻的精神科医生讲述了一个故事：患者 20 岁，是个大学生。有一天人们发现他赤身裸体在河边；声称父亲惩罚了他，而他逃跑了。他被警察送到精神科诊所。有经验的同事诊断他得了精神病并且开了处方药物。案例提供者并不确定，他倾向于相信患者。他想更多了解父子的关系，但是没有机会去找出答案，他报告了案例和他的疑问。

组长是一位有经验的精神科医生。他对小组工作开始的介绍进行干预："我们有一个年轻的案例提供者和一个年轻的患者，案例提供者怀疑父子的冲突。你对此怎么想？"你可以感受到他的干预在引导小组说服案例提供者，有经验的精神科医生是对的。

他倾向于引导组员到一个特定的方向，这样他就限制了组员的想象、自由联想和其他情绪。接下来的讨论，组长强调了支持诊断"精神病"的陈述，忽略了关于父子关系的部分。

幸运的是有一位副组长，他关注了案例提供者并且请他回来，询问了他的感受。案例提供者说："你们多数人都不相信我，但是我确信就是有冲突，也许两者都是真实的。他有精神病，而他的父子关系很糟糕，对他有重要的影响。"

在反馈中，小组和观察者指出了平行进程。案例提供者感到被拒绝，就像那个患者。他有能力表达他的失望，很幸运这里有个副组长能够关注他。

组长很快有了一个假设并试着把小组引导到他的方向。他没有对其他的可能性保持开放。通过反馈，他意识到在讨论中的第一个干预及他的态度限制了这个过程。

组长在培训中得到的反馈取决于作为巴林特小组案例提供者的医生获得了什么：我的情绪如何，我的态度如何影响了关系或小组进程。关于我自己，我的情绪，关于我的偏见、我的投射，我的移情和反移情，我学到了很多。

在这种情况下反馈有助于识别平行进程，在常规巴林特小组中可能不是这样。案例提供者可能会带着这样的感觉回去："也许我错了，但他们并不理解是什么在困扰我，这个巴林特小组没有真正帮到我。"在小组中的经验可能和在诊所一样，他并没有拓宽视野。

在这个培训小组中，现在他了解了，给予抗精神病药物是可以的，同时他想再次和患者交谈，认真对待他并搞清楚他和父亲的关系。

另一个重要的议题是"对小组的问题"。组长倾向于在案例报告结束时问案例提供者："你能给小组提一个问题吗？"这可能会误导小组。向小组提出的问题通常是："这种情况下你会怎么做？"或者"我该怎么对待这个患者？""做"其实是个诱导性的字眼。

在巴林特工作中我们聚焦于移情和反移情，相关的所有情绪、偏见、盲点和无知等，"如何做的问题"背离了小组工作的本质。应该遵循好的建议，实用的贴士，未来处理问题的解决方案。

对于案例提供者有帮助的邀请可以是："你能简要总结一下你和患者的问题吗？""嗯，当我在电脑上看到他的名字时，我已经感觉到不情愿去给他看病，我也不知道为什么。"

鉴于关键问题是关系，通常根本不需要一个问题或总结。"在两个人当中发生了什么？"这始终是小组中的任务。

在有雕塑的巴林特小组中

➤ 案例 10

Frauke，一位年轻的全科医生，报告了一个案例：一对60多岁的老年夫妇进入了她的诊室。老妇人主诉脚肿的鞋都穿不上了。当 Frauke 给她查体时震惊了：她腿上的溃疡往外流脓。查体她的肝脏很硬，腹腔满是腹水。第二天她做了血液检查，如同她所预料的一样，发现了肝硬化的所有症状。其实这对夫妇第一次走进她的诊室，她就闻到了酒味。这时 Frauke 尝试说服他们必须住院进一步诊治，他们拒绝了。患者的母亲下周日过 85 岁生日，而患者承诺过要给她烤个蛋糕，并坚持不能跟母亲说她去不了。Frauke 注意到两人都没有意识到病情有多么严重。他们反复说只想能重新穿上鞋。医生的印象中丈夫是那个阻止她接受诊治的人，她决定下次单独见患者并说服她，她很不喜欢患者丈夫，她想知道怎样

能最好地帮助患者。

组长建议她做个模拟，她同意了：

Susanne：一个在心身诊所工作的医生，扮演患者。

Johannes：在精神科诊所工作，扮演患者丈夫。

Christiane：也在心身诊所工作，扮演医生。

Heike：一个骨科医生，扮演患者 85 岁的母亲。

案例提供者 Frauke 让扮演者站在她认为合适的位置，然后她走到每个人身后给他或她一句话：他（她）在这个位置上的感受或想法。

患者："我不明白自己怎么了，我只想回到以前的样子。"

患者丈夫："我希望你能把她治好。"

母亲："我的生日快到了，我女儿当然会照顾好我。"

医生："我希望帮助她。"

我们知道，这些想法代表了医生对于目前情况的内在设想。这是我们的机会，去改变焦点，从而创造其他可能性，照亮盲点。

Frauke 这位案例提供者现在从远处看着这个场景。"遮挡眼睛的第一片叶子"落下了，突然理解了患者的处境和她自己的情绪反应。

设计显示，母亲、丈夫和医生把患者往不同方向引导。

下一步是询问扮演者他们在自己位置上的感受，以及他们想做什么改变。

访问扮演者是组长的任务。重要的是使用开放式问题，而不指向某个答案。

组长问："在这个位置你感觉怎么样？"而不是，"这难道不是个困难处境吗？你不是应该更好地为了健康而照顾自己吗？"这类的封闭式问题，患者只能选择说"是"或"否"。

患者回答了这个开放式问题，她感到有压力，不知道该相

信谁，该听谁的。她没有把疾病当回事。她的肚子肿胀和脚肿胀令她很困扰，她只想把这些症状治好恢复更好的功能。她的问题是：她无法照顾丈夫和母亲，她希望和医生及丈夫坐下来讨论下一步怎么办。

对于丈夫，一个可能的封闭式问题是："你没看见妻子病有多严重吗？"

而开放式问题："你的感觉是什么？"这可以获得更多信息。

丈夫感到烦恼和愤怒，因为日常生活被干扰了，妻子不在家只剩他自己，因为她得了病。他想把妻子带走，把医生和母亲甩到身后。他更相信自己的经验，认为酒精总能解决所有的问题，而不是医生。

对于母亲，一个可能的封闭式问题是："你是否意识到女儿的问题？"

对于开放式问题："你感觉怎么样？"她回答，她看到女儿背对着她，还有医生在房间里，感到不安。她希望女儿看着她这边，只是关注她而不是别人。

医生表达了她的不舒服，她想和患者单独相处，把母亲和丈夫排除在外。

Frauke 作为案例提供者仔细地听。

这时组长请她决定谁可以有机会改变结局。

Frauke 说："患者可以改变。"

第二个模拟：这是患者创造的——患者，她的丈夫和医生呈三角形坐在一起。以下是组长用开放式问题采访的答案：患者看不到她的母亲，她感到放松了。新的场景中医生也感觉更好。患者丈夫并不满意但能够接受这个改变。患者母亲感到生气、失望和焦虑。

之后小组像往常一样进入小组讨论。形象设计大概花

10～15分钟，而我们总是需要90分钟进行一个案例的工作。如果有两个组长，让另一位组长组织讨论可能是个明智之选，他可以从远处看到案例设计而不进入场景当中。

他可以先问案例提供者："经历了模拟，你对小组的问题有改变吗？"

或者他可以从对于小组的干预开始："你们记得这个故事，也参与了模拟过程，对于医患关系有哪些感受、想法或想象？"

此后小组的讨论很活跃，没有给予理智化建议。可以感受到而不仅是考虑到情绪。

当然，我们聚焦在医患关系上，组长只是偶尔提醒一下小组。

Frauke 对于她的关系有了一个不同的视角。她明白，去说服患者并不一定要和母亲和丈夫去争，因为她已经能够从另一个角度看这个场景，她感到自己的要求不现实。现在她可以接受这个状况了，接受它的存在并争取最好的结果。她感受到悲伤并看到一线希望。

她印象深刻，甚至她对患者丈夫的感受也在这个过程中改变了。他的存在不再困扰她，她表达了对于再次见到患者的好奇心。

这个模拟也有不利的一面。

Johannes，那个年轻的精神科医生，因为他的感受而惊讶，在患者丈夫的角色中，他没有意识到酒精对于自己和伴侣的损害作用，因为没有人能够告诉他这一点。

在现实生活中，他作为精神科医生试图说服他的患者，酒精和药物对于精神和身体的负面影响，如果成瘾者不听从他的观点，他常感到失望。在模拟中他也感受到了否认。

Susanne，作为患者，意识到她对于接受严重疾病的抵触。她必须迎合她的母亲和丈夫，而他们也否认她的病，对她而言这是个新的经验。

Christiane，作为医生，对这种情况感到紧张、恐惧和愤怒。同时她希望能提供帮助，然而她没有成功。她的第一个想法：戒掉酒精，彻底改变生活，摆脱你的依赖，而她明白对于这个患者而言是不可能的，这个家庭和她自己有着完全不同的生活世界、生活目标和方向。这是给患者传递一个属于她的信息——巴林特称之为"使命"，"意思是每个医生都应该有一个坚定的信念：当患者生病时应该如何应对。"（Balint，1957 年）

在模拟中每个扮演者都产生了强烈的情绪，既获得了共情又有每个人的自我经验，不一定要用语言表达出来，但会留在他们心里。

在后续的讨论中我们会使用他们的情绪体验来更好地了解情况。

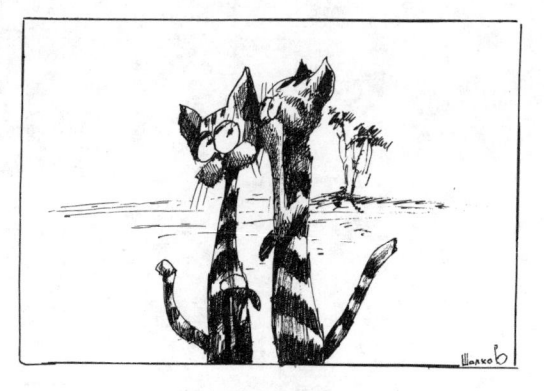

医生给患者的信息

当然，旁观者们也会在讨论中加入他们的观察所见和情绪。

组长的任务是使用这些情绪来表达，帮助扮演者们回到元位置，聚焦医患关系及其外部影响因素。

我们知道场景的设置来源于案例提供者的感知。它是主观的，

反映了患者和他们的生活体系所唤起的案例提供者的情绪。

模拟提供了一个与现实交流的机会，打开不同的观点和新的想法，在一个健康的距离下，带着微笑和幽默回来——尽管在案例中、在工作环境中、在医疗保健系统中仍有着各种困难。

几周后这个小组再次相聚，组长询问有什么反馈。Frauke 说她非常惊讶，那位患者下一次就诊时没有和丈夫一起来。她衣着讲究、干净，没有酒味。这就像个奇迹"好像当时听到了小组讨论……"Frauke 觉得好奇并很开心地见到患者。她能够支持患者可以有各种可能性，就像小组能够支持她——这不是用"好的建议"或道德约束来强迫她。

09 带领不同的小组

有一位受认证的组长曾经对我说："培训以外带领小组工作比我想象的要困难得多，那和在组长工作坊的体会大相径庭。"确实如此。在组长工作坊，你和非常有经验的同事一起工作，他们已经经过心理学思维的培训。在现实世界中，小组工作面对的是某种意义上的"门外汉"，而巴林特的目标，用他的话来讲是："带着心理思维行医"。作为组长，我们的工作是帮助从业者，他们大多数不习惯用分析性的思维去考虑医患关系。

同质性和异质性的小组

巴林特在伦敦开创了全科医生的小组。第二次世界大战后，他受邀帮助他们了解有心身反应的患者。巴林特和他的第一任妻子爱丽丝在匈牙利布达佩斯已经有过和小组工作的经验。现在他想传授心身医学，同时研究"医生"这种药物的药理学。他称自己的小组为"训练暨研究小组"。训练医生的心身医学知识、诊断和治疗，已经能更好地了解医生对于他的患者所起的作用，医患关系对于诊断和治疗的影响。"医生即是药物"。

在只有全科医生组成的小组工作既有优点，也有缺点。同一个职业的组员有着大量相同的经历。你不需要解释家访的困难或者不依从患者带着新的主诉反复上门，因为他们都知道。另一方面，你们的想法可能都朝着一个方向，而其他专业的人可能从别的角度看问题更能发现盲点。同质小组可能有着同样的心理防御。

巴林特的想法是讨论全科医生在日常行医中的心理学潜意识。

他作为精神科医生了解更多心身疾病的背景和心身互动，但他并不想去教育这个小组，他希望全科医生发现潜在的问题，就像是心理治疗师并没有对来访者进行教育，但是帮助他理解了自己的内在冲突。

在同质小组中，组员对于如何面对患者和机构有着类似的经历和困难。他们的职业认同、自我形象和自我了解也相似。这些可能有助于投入案例和医生的需要，但这也可能唤起共同的防御。由于他们的工作经历和医疗环境相似，特定患者的个体问题和患者的观点容易被投射到这些环境当中。这样自我体验部分被丢弃并限制了新的视角，而参与者们就不会像在研究项目中所发现的那样获得自我成长，除非组长像巴林特那样，是一位有心理治疗背景的专家。他就会指出和引导参与者去了解个体的冲突。一个同质的小组可能一致认为应该强迫她去做，并考虑怎么才能成功做到。当组长邀请案例提供者回来而且她能够表达受挫感后小组工作才得以推进。此后平行进程让某些人进入患者的角色。"没人知道我的慢性病是多大的负担。"这对一个在日常工作中不面对同样问题的成员更为容易。在同质小组中，组长经常需要把话题转到患者的角度。而在不同专业背景的异质小组中这个可能性更小。可能有批判性的反思，局外人的观点常有帮助。患者的视角更容易出现。

异质小组的缺点是，有更多的误解需要去澄清，但有时这些问题也可以更好地带来新想法，启发案例提供者，而且其他专业领域的人认为很有趣。

对于巴林特小组组长最重要的是有足够的能力在这些领域了解案例提供者和组员们的理性和非理性的发言。

医生、心理学家、精神科医生的小组

混合小组带来不同角度的立场和有意思的观点。对于案例提供

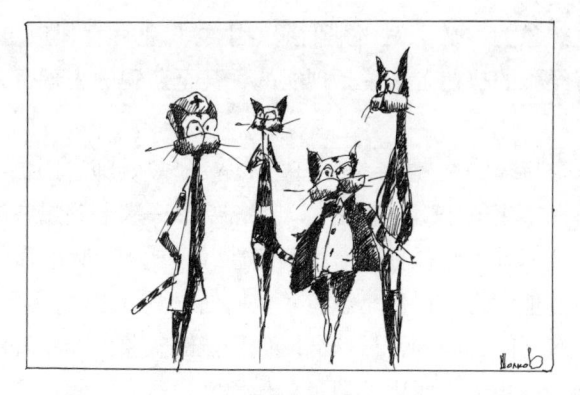

混合小组

者的故事，不同人物的观点是多样化的。当不在同一个专业，似乎更容易站在患者和家属的立场去看问题。一个精神科医生的观点与全科医生或妇科医生或学生会有所不同。我们经常体会到，当你还不明白和其他人，如患者之间发生了什么就生气了。当你找到了合理的解释，愤怒消失了。共情是这种理解的重要前提。在一个不同的人、不同的患者和不同故事的小组中，你的共情可以得到更好的训练。

混合小组的组长会从其他专业人士那里学到很多。这培养了他的开放、宽容、尊重和好奇心。作为组长你已经知道在小组中和不同领域的专家一起工作，你是小组动力和分析性思维的专家，组员们则是各自领域的专家。

学生的小组

最初巴林特不想将学生纳入小组。他认为他们不够成熟，无法在医患关系的问题上与其他组员产生共鸣。最终是 Boris Luban-Plozza 说服了他，学生们有自己的观点，而且尚未被常规和挫折所破坏，这对于小组工作有启发性的影响。他们能够自由联想，有新

点子，让想象力绽放。对于他们期望中的职业常有理想化的观点，这对于有经验的执业者来说是现实的，甚至悲观的表现带来有价值的一面。

在医生与医学生的混合小组中，大家可以从彼此身上学到很多。

只有医学生的小组也很完美。通常给第一次遇到患者的学生带来安慰，他们并不是孤单面对不确定性、挣扎和批评。医学生还不是医生，但他们也不仅仅是患者。他们处于两者之间。当他们描述自己与患者之间的问题常被认同。他们能够想象一个年轻的临终患者或意外伤的患者，医生的角色对他们来说还有些陌生和不安，并非常规和完全接受。对于医疗体制、医疗实践和医疗保险的批判也值得一听，还有如何改进医学生培训。

▶ 案例 11

两名医学院 3 年级的学生在外科病房实习，按要求他们要在患者手术前采集病史和体格检查，他们一起在医院房间的门外等候。一个外科医生经过问他们："你们在找什么？——哦，对不起，我忘了，你们要到这里检查患者。我现在没时间，请在这里等着。"1 小时以后："哦，你们还在这。没有人带你们看病人吗？我会派人来做。"又 1.5 小时过去了："快来，我会快速让你们见到患者。我知道你们的研讨会时间都过了。"他们进入一个房间。一位 70 岁的患者面色苍白、焦虑地躺在床上。医生快速走过去，移走他的毯子，指着他的腹部，并请学生们观察和检查。学生们犹豫了，他们觉得羞愧。他们怎能就这样接触病人呢？"我是 Frank，对不起，我能看吗？我能接触你的身体吗？"患者安静点头。Frank 检查触到上腹部一个大肿瘤。"现在这是什么？"外科医生不耐烦地问。"我触到上腹部肿瘤"。"是的，正确，这个患者得了胰腺癌。我们明天手术。机会不大，但我们会尽力。你们可以明天来看手术。我得

走了。如果你们还有时间，可以和这个患者谈谈，询问他的病史。无论如何我都会给你们签字的。明天见。"这两个学生听了都很震惊，他们看到患者眼中有泪。该怎么办呢？"我们能问您一些问题吗？还是您想独处？"Frank 问。"谢谢你问我，不过我希望一个人。"他们两个带着糟糕的心情离开了。

小组感到感动、愤怒、激动。多数人马上进入患者的角色，其他人表达了对 Frank 的共情。真是个糟糕的状况。此前有人跟这个患者谈过吗？还是他一直都被这样对待？怎么能如此残忍？为什么医学生被这样对待？他们感到累赘、无用、多余，但他们是未来的医生。为什么现在的医生不愿意尽最大努力教授他们的知识呢？他们知道一个外科医生的任务多么繁重和令人疲劳，但这能成为如此对待患者和医学生的借口吗？Frank 感到被接纳和理解后好多了。小组里的所有学生都表示今后在他们的职业生涯中，会用不同的方式对待这类情况，也希望他们能记住这次巴林特小组。

重要的一点是，要更好地学习如何与患者交谈并听取他们的故事。

对于组长而言，重要的是了解医学生在巴林特小组中讨论会遇到什么样的困难。

我们在还有 1 年大学毕业的医学生中发现了 4 个重复出现的巴林特工作主题：

① 医学生在医学训练中的自我社会化问题。

② 医学生在教学医院中的临床工作中角色。

③ 理想的医生形象和现实的冲突。

④ 自我体验的愿望和需要。

带领医学生的巴林特小组具有一些独特之处。作为医生或者心理学家的组长，常被看作是诊所或者医疗机构的代表或是简单理性

躯体医学的反对者。有时却被理想化地视为一个知道自己所有情绪反应和可能性，又能同时用整体视角照顾好患者的身体和情绪需要的医生。

在巴林特小组中，医学生努力处理他们日常临床工作，常感到经验不足。一段时间后，他们变得更宽容、更现实，对于患者的理想化的和现实的方法有了更为多样化的图像。重点是需要包含两个方面：理性和情绪，躯体和心理。

这个组长想起了他自己在学生时代的努力。这可能是在教学和体验中保持平衡的优势。

国际巴林特联盟（IBF）和心身医学和社会医学基金会联合设立了一项每两年评选一次的奖学金，支持世界各地的医学生和他们的文章，叙述医患关系，他们对此的思考以及医学教育和医疗系统的思考。过去近40年的医学生的文章有一部分已经出版了。这些对于不同国家这些年医学生在医学培训中的经验提供了有益的资料。

其他助人工作者的小组

我们提及不同职业各种助人者的小组，如医生、心理学家、护士、社工、运动治疗师、医学助理、物理治疗师、音乐治疗师、医院的牧师、教师。这些小组的前提和共识是每个参与者都愿意分享他们自己困难的关系故事，并真正参与解决的过程。另一个重要的议题是保密：小组中所说的所有内容留在小组里，不在其他地方讨论。

小组成员从他们各自领域的真实经历及不同的视角能够为解决问题和启发带来潜在贡献。

对于不同领域人员的巴林特小组，组长需要宽容、尊重和了解不同的领域，这对他自己的职业既是挑战也是充实。

不同文化背景和国籍

时至今日，巴林特小组中有不同文化背景的成员已成为家常便饭。同时，报告的患者也来自不同国家。作为巴林特小组组长，你很幸运小组中有成员可以解释由于这种背景带来的某些行为、信念、典型的焦虑。正如巴林特说的："组长不应该是小组中最聪明的人"。他收集发言并发现其价值，作为组长你从组员那里学到很多，欢迎偏见并使它们开放。这样你就可以发现自己的错误。"老师都是思想狭隘的""所有的乡下人都是天真的"等等，你会在小组中发现很多例子，明智的做法是思考自己作为组长的偏见并去修正它们。

➤ 案例 12

这是在精神科诊所内精神科医生培训的巴林特小组。这也是他们成为专科医生必须训练的一部分。小组成员来自俄罗斯、乌克兰、土耳其、伊朗、波兰和德国。

一名土耳其学员报告案例：患者是 43 岁男性，在土耳其的村庄长大，18 岁到了德国并从那时起在包办婚姻中生活。他在一家小公司当技术工人。他有两个女儿，分别为 16 岁和 18 岁。他形容自己结婚后很有攻击性，经常和妻子吵架并打过她，不经常在家，花了很多钱赌博，不照顾他的孩子。父亲 2009 年去世，他突然非常害怕。他转向宗教，到麦加做了朝圣。回来后变成了好父亲、好丈夫，定期去做祈祷。他的生活彻底改变了。7 年后他因为抑郁来到精神科诊所。他说最近两年饱受内心不安、睡眠障碍和焦虑的折磨。他母亲 2013 年去世时他精神崩溃了。从那以后他看到不同的人物，他称为"吉恩"（Dschinn），决定他的生活事务。他们就在那里，他能看

见他们，他们告诉他做什么。他不敢违背，那些吉恩有的和善，有的折磨他。

案例提供者来自土耳其，他成长中也有"吉恩"。他向小组解释，他们相信有超自然的生物和我们一起生活，只是我们一般看不见，只有在特殊情况下他们才能看得见。他小时候，大人告诫他："小心，'吉恩'看着并知道你做的一切。现在他不知道该怎么想。这个患者是偏执吗？或者是魔法想象？他曾经试图说服患者，"吉恩"只是他的想象，虽然他在情感上不是那么确定，但在理智上是肯定的。患者很固执，而且抗精神病药物也没有帮助。案例提供者感到无助和不确定。

在小组讨论中，来自不同文化背景的成员很快就把患者看作是一个小男孩。他们有一些想象的画面，如一个坏人在床底下，一个天使在上面。父母支持那些好的天使。他们照顾你、保护你，他们永远和你在一起，而坏人只是想象，但坏的角色也是必要的。有时父母用这样的画面：坏人在树林里，会来抓走淘气的孩子，或者圣诞老人，给好人礼物，打坏人。所有文化都有类似的故事。

坏的角色在某方面是有帮助的，它们接管了攻击性的情绪和欲望。不是那个小男孩掐了他弟弟，弄坏了他心爱的泰迪熊的耳朵，偷了他姐姐的巧克力棒——是那个淘气的角色。我们需要花一段时间去整合我们讨厌的部分，这个患者可能没有整合它们，他压抑或者分裂了所有和他的新宗教生活不相称的情绪。他用"吉恩"把不想要的情绪转移给了它们。案例提供者有点怀疑，但还是带走了新的想法。医患关系像一个父亲和5岁的男孩吗？那是移情和反移情吗？

6周后案例提供者反馈：他改变了对这个患者的设计，他们散步、讨论政治和其他现实世界的事实问题。他们更多把目光转向这个层面。患者在这个层面对争论保持开放，可以理解

他的处境。他对"吉恩"谈得不多，但当他提到它们，他不再焦虑了。当它们嘲笑他，他会想："等着瞧，我会成功的。"精神科医生的印象是患者更为成熟和进步，可以和他孩子式地想象拉开一定距离，而医生自己更像是一个伙伴，而不是以前那个父亲。

在结构化和放手之间，不同小组的不同风格

我曾经与很多不同构成的小组开展过工作：医学生、全科医生、精神科医生、妇科医生、教授、年轻医生、混合小组、心身医学基本培训的小组、周末工作坊小组、经验丰富和无经验的，在中国，在俄罗斯，在罗马尼亚等等，在国际会议、IBF 大会上等，我不会说自己一直是同一个组长。我根据自己推进小组的印象行事。

我的主要问题是："这个小组需要在多大程度上结构化？"

自由联想和想象需要空间。有经验的小组应该有大的空间，他们不需要太多口头干预；组长常用肢体语言。他们需要安全的气氛、细心的支持和明确的时间框架。

没有经验的小组需要更多干预。有时干预可以是一个解释或一个问题或一个挑战以打开新的方向，不需要纠正或评价发言。对参与者提问可以启发场景画面。"你为什么这么想？"或者"你的话背后是什么？""你的感受是什么？"回答经常是"我想……"而组长再次问："你的感受是什么？"尤其是医生群体已经被训练得理性，当然对于日常工作很有意义。把这种习惯转换到另一个角度并不容易。

医学生经常随时敞开谈论他们的情绪、他们的个人生活、他们的背景，在这里需要限制开放程度以保护个体。

有时在长期工作的巴林特小组也会如此。它越来越向自我体验

小组发展。常年累月组员们彼此熟悉，可能有私人接触，从同一个人那里听到了很多类似的医患关系故事。这时可能这个同事的困难已经很明显了，他和什么样的患者相处有问题，这可能使得小组难以对新思想保持开放。小组可能发展出共同的防御和共同的盲点。希望组长不要和他们一起，继续保持从元位置看问题。

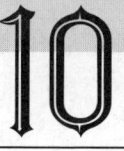

10　巴林特小组组长的督导

　　我们大多数人都希望和其他的组长交流思想、谈谈某个组员的困难、小组处境的困难、困难的事件或者两位组长之间的冲突，而且这种交谈愿望不仅限于在开始做组长的阶段。也许有人想知道如何建立一个新的小组，以此与其他组长多交流。

　　巴林特小组组长的问题是：可以在哪里寻求帮助呢？当然，给另一位组长打电话是可以的，或首先和副组长讨论这个问题。

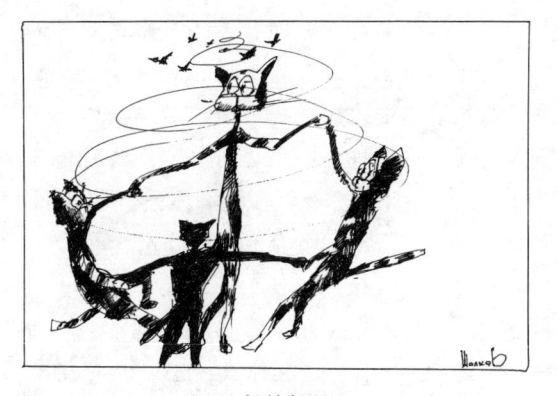

组长的督导

有主持人的督导小组

　　经常参加巴林特小组组长的督导对小组是有帮助的。这些督导小组通常有一个主持人组织协调。你可以像自我体验小组一样工作或像巴林特小组报告"患者"一样报告（讲述）一个小组或者组

员的故事。这时就有了一个故事，提问环节和讨论，可以用自由联想、想象和认同开展工作。就像在医患关系中一样，你可能在报告的组长－案例提供者关系中发现盲点。

▶ **案例 13**

　　6个有经验的巴林特小组组长在一个督导的主持下坐在一起，他们决定采用一个巴林特小组似的设置：他们中的一位报告案例，其他人先仔细听，然后他们可以提问澄清性问题，然后报告者后退，过一会儿再回来。

　　一位成员报告了他在精神科诊所的一个小组。由12位成员组成，但通常6~8人出席，很少达到10人。他们都是培训中的精神科医生。这个小组在每天结束的时候工作，一半是工作时间，一半是他们的自由时间。参与者常是疲惫的，但他们喜欢用想象、思考、幽默和笑声开展巴林特小组工作。唯一让组长恼怒的是组员不能准时。他理解有时候难以遵守时间，但他对此很不高兴。他和这个小组之间出了什么问题？

　　督导小组的多数参与者对此都很熟悉。临床医生总是很忙，他们会匆匆走进小组，甚至在小组工作中睡着。他们一天看很多患者，夜间还要值班。他们一边接受培训一边参加其他的课程和会议。主持人说他们都很善解人意，只有对年轻同事的共情吗？有人说："不，这也让我愤怒。我希望我的巴林特小组值得让他们从头到尾享受其中。"另外有人说："我必须每天工作，而且我总是守时，为什么他们不行？"讨论现在沿着这个方向进行。他们自己接受培训的回忆浮现出来，那时他们必须严格遵守规定。当然他们有时痛恨规定并想逃走。

　　报告者突然说："哦，我希望小组爱我！我很慷慨，想像个好父亲一样在艰苦工作之余给他们快乐，但我没有给他们足够的界限，这是他们在工作生活的平衡中非常需要的。我应

该在提出要求方面成为更好的榜样，而不是在他们面前掩饰愤怒。"然后参与者讨论了他们将如何告诉这个小组。愤怒已经在他们发现后就消失了。也许你会问这个小组组员的相互支持，有人总是准时，组长总是准时，他们怎么做到的？他们所有人一起开始的益处是什么？

督导小组大多在周末工作坊会面，他们为新思路和改变提供了一个机会。通常是没有反馈的。无论如何在团体中讨论这些困难可以是一种释放，并得到不同观点和支持。就像在常规巴林特小组中一样影响是多方面的；每个人都有类似的经历。

参加者也可以讨论一般性问题，如：你怎么建立一个新的小组？你会提供茶或咖啡吗？这对小组工作可能有什么影响？在巴林特小组中你会拒绝讨论什么？你是怎么做的？如果一个组员在过程中离开，要做什么？当你发现了问题是否会在小组后和这个组员谈谈？如何处理一个对你带领小组有压力的情况？

更多的问题可能会随之而来，如果能够交流它们就很好。

内视团体

另一种可能性是我们所称的"内视团体"。组长们聚在一起讨论他们的小组，不设主持人。

这两种方法都可以帮助组长提高组长工作的质量。

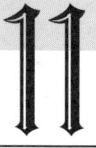

11 组长的任务

通用任务

① 创造安全的氛围；

② 聚焦医患关系；

③ 鼓励思考、想象、自由联想、表达情绪和身体感觉、对话、情景画面、角色扮演；

④ 提供对于现场冲突、小组进程和平行进程的解释；

⑤ 区分案例的动力与小组的动力，尤其是紧急的外来干扰因素；

⑥ 觉察自己的情绪，移情和反移情；

⑦ 激发新的视角；

⑧ 激发共情和兴趣。

带模拟小组中的任务

① 他像常规小组一样开场；

② 在澄清性问题之后，他请案例提供者选择人物扮演者；

③ 他协助做模拟；

④ 他访问模拟中的人物；

⑤ 他请案例提供者选择模拟中改变的人；

⑥ 他再次访问人物；

⑦ 他或副组长主持后续讨论。

组长遵守模拟的目的

① 通过使用肢体语言达到情绪水平；

② 使得医患关系和他们所工作和生活的系统可视化，可被觉察；

③ 通过工作拓宽案例提供者的视野；

④ 激发新的观点；

⑤ 帮助案例提供者放松；

⑥ 重新获得对患者的兴趣；

⑦ 提升行医的乐趣。

组长意识到的副作用

① 几乎每个组员都经历过类似的困难患者或处境；

② 过程中被唤起的情绪留存并可被回忆；

③ 对于模拟中人物的认同有自我体验的一面，这部分自然发生，不加讨论；

④ 模拟的形象留在脑海中并影响医患沟通；

⑤ 扮演者可能有一些不能与小组分享的自我体验。

12 结 论

听起来当巴林特小组的组长真是令人精疲力尽。

但好消息是,当小组工作时组长有时间反思。

我们的小组通常用 90 分钟处理一个案例中的医患关系。

这给予了仔细倾听、案例提供者和小组,从情绪水平转到元位置再回来的可能性。

当小组开始工作,组长可以关注自己的情绪并形成自己关于医患关系的假设。

同时他听取小组的讨论并观察案例提供者的反应。

就像在心理治疗中我们的移情和反移情,共情和情绪反应是作为组长工作的工具。

这就是为什么在开始组长培训之前希望能有自我体验,因为我们是和小组一起工作,了解团体动力也是必要的。

13 国际巴林特联盟——巴林特小组组长认证标准

这些标准旨在供各国巴林特协会设计他们的认证标准时参考。例如，各国协会希望定义成为巴林特小组组长足够的时间周期。各协会组织需要了解精神科医生和心理治疗师在认证前有带领巴林特小组的经验同样重要，全科医生也是如此，而精神科医生和心理治疗师与全科医生的路径会有所不同。

1）组长需要有适当的基础职业培训。

2）组长必须有参加巴林特小组的前期经验，时间足够*。

3）作为组长培训的一部分，组长需要与有资质的组长共同带组，并向认证协会提交书面报告（证明信）。

4）组长应该接受足够的有资质督导者**的工作督导，并向认证协会提供书面报告／证明信。

5）组长认证前需要根据以下标准接受评估：

① 他们鼓励发展安全和自由的小组环境，了解保护小组边界的重要性；

② 他们的工作聚焦于探索医患关系而非寻求答案或教学；

③ 他们对学习带领小组的个人风格保持开放，并意识到他们的态度和反应将影响小组的动力；

④ 他们能意识到可能影响小组主要任务的小组进程和无意识过程；

⑤ 他们认识到成为受认证的巴林特小组组长是个开始而非结束；

6）组长应当接受充分的持续性督导。

* 由认证协会决定

** 在某些协会可能目前达不到

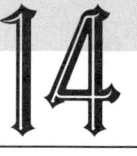

14 德国的巴林特小组组长认证标准

临床医生必须满足的要求

① 德国巴林特协会成员，至少在最近 1 次巴林特小组组长研讨会入会；

② 开始组长培训时缴纳 100 欧元注册费；

③ 另外的专业培训包括：心理治疗或精神分析或特殊的心理治疗医学或心身医学或精神科与心理治疗或儿童青少年精神科与心理治疗；

④ 在完成以上培训后在该领域工作 3 年。在这 3 年中参加巴林特小组，可以是德国巴林特协会认证组长带领的连续性小组或者德国巴林特协会举办的周末工作坊，至少参加 70 次小组活动；

⑤ 如果没有参加第 3 条中专业培训中的巴林特小组训练，必须参加另外 35 次德国巴林特协会认证组长带领的连续性小组；

⑥ 参加 6 次巴林特小组组长研讨会，至少参加 30 个单元由德国巴林特协会认证的培训师指导的培训。其中至少 4 次研讨会应为德国巴林特协会举办的工作坊。在这些研讨会中必须完成至少 2 次督导下的带领小组工作；

⑦ 须有在连续性小组或工作坊中做副组长的经验；

⑧ 认证由德国巴林特联盟委员会及培训委员会共同做出；

⑨ 可以在德国巴林特协会（网址：www.balintgesellschaft.de）的首页上下载表格，填写并提交。

心理学家必须满足的要求

① 有资质的心理学家并接受其他的心理治疗或精神分析培训；

② 在完成其他培训后在心理治疗或精神分析专业工作 3 年；

③ 参加 105 次德国巴林特协会认证组长带领的巴林特小组；

④ 至少上述 35 次为连续性小组；

⑤ 参加 6 次巴林特小组组长研讨会，至少参加 30 个单元由德国巴林特协会认证的培训师指导的培训，其中至少 4 次研讨会应为德国巴林特协会举办的工作坊，在这些研讨会中必须完成至少 2 次督导下的带领小组工作；

⑥ 德国巴林特协会成员，至少在最近 1 次巴林特小组组长研讨会入会；

⑦ 须有在连续性小组或工作坊中做副组长的经验；

⑧ 认证由德国巴林特联盟委员会及培训委员会共同做出；

⑨ 缴纳认证费 100 欧元；

⑩ 可以在德国巴林特协会（网址：www.balintgesellschaft.de）的首页上下载表格，填写并提交。

15 参 考 文 献

Balint M (1972) The Doctor, His Patient and the Illness, International Universities Press, Inc. , New York

Flatten G, Möller H, Tschuschke V (2015) Designing the doctor-patient relationship - How beneficial are Balint groups and for whom? Proceedings of the 1st International Balint Conference, Yerevan

Otten H (2012) Professionelle Beziehungen. Springer, Berlin Heidelberg

Otten H, Petzold ER (2015) The Student, the Patient and the Illness 2015, Berlin

Petzold ER, Otten H (2010) The Student, the Patient and the Illness, Xlibri